Your Quest for Home

A Guidebook to Find the Ideal Community for Your Later Years

By

Marianne Kilkenny

Marianne Kilkenny

NOTICE: You Do NOT Have the Right to Reprint or Resell this Guidebook

You Also **MAY NOT** Give Away, Sell or Share the Content Herein

ALL RIGHTS RESERVED. No part of this Guidebook or series may be reproduced or transmitted in any form whatsoever, electronic, or mechanical, including photocopying, recording, or by any informational storage or retrieval system, without the express written, dated and signed permission of the authors.

With one exception: You have my permission to photocopy the exercises for your own personal use and use with those whom you want to share Community.

DISCLAIMER AND/OR LEGAL NOTICES

The information presented herein represents the view of the authors as of the date of publication. Because of the rate with which conditions change, the authors reserve the right to alter and update their opinions based on— new conditions. The publication is for informational purposes only. While every attempt has been made to verify the information provided in this publication, neither the authors nor their affiliates/partners assume any responsibility for errors, inaccuracies or omissions. Any slights of people or organizations are unintentional. If advice concerning legal or related matters is needed, the services of a fully qualified professional should be sought. This publication is not intended for use as a source of legal business practices in your country or state. Any reference to any person or business, whether living or dead, is purely coincidental.

DEDICATION

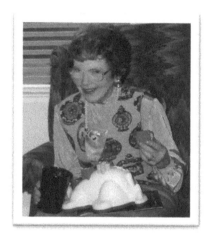

To my mom, Betty Jane Martin, who was a woman before her time. She was my hero and she continues inspiring me to find new ways to help others to age with grace and dignity.

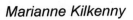

Marianne Kilkenny

CONTENTS

WHO NEEDS THIS GUIDEBOOK

Chances are if you have picked up this Guidebook you are wondering if living in Community is right for you. Or at the very least, you have wondered what it's all about.

This Guidebook begins to answer that question for you. It will also help you define what kind of Community would meet your needs and assists you to go out there and create it.

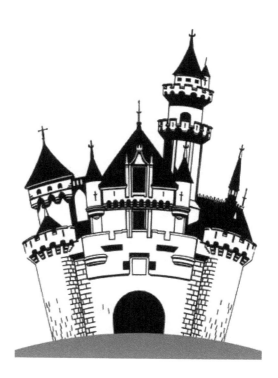

1

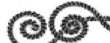
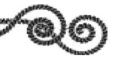

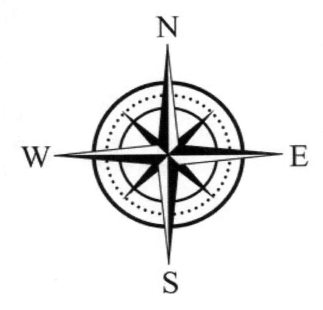

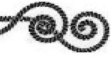

WHY I WROTE THIS GUIDEBOOK

It was my real honor to be with my parents as they aged and their lives drew to an end. They were independent and proud people. But despite having two loving and attentive daughters who lived nearby, they were unable to bypass having to live in a nursing home. It was not the way any of us had envisioned their last years.

Experiencing this with my parents caused me to fear my own aging and final years. But unlike my parents, I had no spouse or children to lean on. I began to fret about what would happen to me. I was determined to find an alternative to the nursing home. This fear, and my desire to find a better way, was the beginning of my Quest—my Quest to find new and different ways to age gracefully.

That was many years and many workshops, seminars, and conversations ago, all bringing me to the point of writing this Guidebook. My hope is that you find this Guidebook a helpful resource, a time-saver and a companion as you work to find your Happily Ever After.

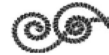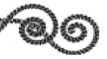

"In and through
community lies the salvation
of the world."
Scott Peck

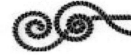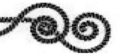

SECTION 1

YOUR PERSONAL JOURNEY

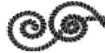
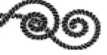

Marianne Kilkenny

"Twenty years from
now you will be
more disappointed
by the things you
didn't do than by
the ones you did."
                    Mark Twain

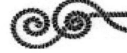
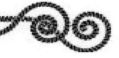

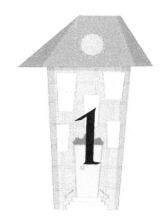

HOW TO USE THIS GUIDEBOOK

If you bought this Guidebook then it is likely you are on a Quest. A Quest to define and find where you want to live and, perhaps more importantly, how you want to live.

Like all Quests, it will not always be straightforward. There will be some twists and turns, some unexpected obstacles and perhaps even times when you wish you had never started out on it at all.

Hi, I'm the Grand Nudge. I'm here to encourage and even push you to make time to find your Happily Ever After. I think you're worth it! (I know I am). I don't want you to have this Guidebook and a dream for community and put both of them on the shelf. I believe in you and I'm here to help!

That is where this Guidebook comes in. I have assembled tools here to help you find your way. It's a sort of map, yet where it leads will be totally up to you.

Trust you are meant to be on this journey. Carry this book along as your guide and believe that you will find your Happily Ever After.

7

"One of the oldest human needs is having someone to wonder where you are when you don't come home at night."

Margaret Mead

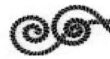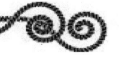

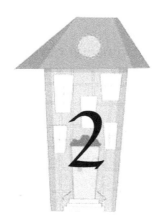

WHAT'S IN YOUR KNAPSACK?

Let's talk about the kinds of things you need as you begin your journey.

The Guidebook:

This Guidebook is filled with information but it also has places for you to take notes, make summaries of the material and record your feelings. In other words, chronicle your journey. We call these sections the Travel Log. You can use the Travel Log sections or your own journal; either way I highly recommend you make notes.

A Notebook or Binder

You will be collecting information all along the way and you need somewhere to put it. Equally as important as collecting it, you need to be able to reference it from time to time. This is why I like a 3-ring binder. I find it more versatile than a spiral notebook. In a 3-ring binder you can add things and move things around as needed. I also use the clear plastic sleeves that have 3 holes in them so I can add pictures and miscellaneous odd-shaped items in my notebook.

Blank Journal

This is optional, but there are going to be many times in this Guidebook when I suggest you write down or journal some things. You can do it in the Guidebook (I've given you plenty of space) but some people find it easier to have a blank journal to record all of their thoughts in one place.

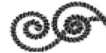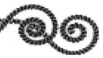

Cork Board on the Wall

If you are a visual person, you might consider having a place on a wall in your home to pin up pictures, ideas or your to-do list.

Computer File

Internet research will be a part of your journey, so before you get into your research I recommend setting up a file folder to keep all your goodies. There are excellent ways to do this with Evernote®, Dropbox®, the Cloud® and others being developed all the time. You might even set up a bookmark file in your browser to save all the cool websites you find. The key here is making it easy to go back to things that you find. I suggest you save things along the way.

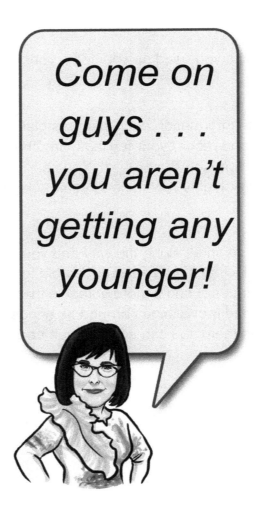

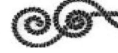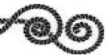

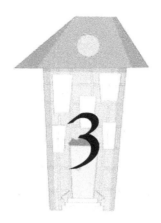

COMMITMENT

Every program works best when you are truly committed to it. Please take some time to read through the following statements. When you feel you can commit to each one of these, please sign the page at the bottom.

- I commit to reading this Guidebook by _____.
- I agree to complete each exercise.
- I will make defining and then creating my Community a priority.
- I will make a schedule for doing this work and then keep to it. (i.e. 1 hour each morning, Sunday afternoons, etc.)
- I understand that this may take longer than I imagine.
- I will take time to reflect on what I learn about myself and seek outside help to move through roadblocks if and when they arise.
- If possible, I will find someone who will take this Quest with me.
- I will celebrate my successes.
- I will allow myself to transform through this process.
- I give myself permission to not do this perfectly, but to the best of my ability.

_____   _____

Signature   Date

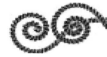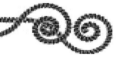

"There are people who make things happen, those who watch what happens and those who wonder what happened."

Unknown

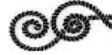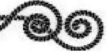

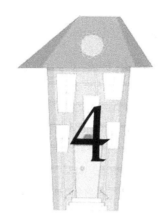

DOES THIS SOUND FAMILIAR?

I'm not sure anyone can escape those pesky, worrisome thoughts about getting older. Most all of us worry about things like: Will we be healthy as we age? Will our money hold out? Will we have people in our lives to help us when and if we need it?

Society (at least our mainstream American one) has some unhealthy assumptions about aging as well. As a member of this society, we may adopt some of these assumptions such as:

- All people get frail and sick as they age.
- "I'm going to be well until the day I die".
- At some time, we all get carted off to a nursing home.
- All retirement is the same.
- Our kids will take care of us.
- Someone/Government is going to build places or fix this problem.

But we know these assumptions aren't necessarily true. There is evidence all over the place that many of us are aging amazingly well, a nursing home is not in our future nor do we want it to be, and our kids . . . if we have them . . . have their own lives.

These overarching messages and fear can collide with what we are truly experiencing or what we can create. The danger is in the old adage of self-fulfilling prophecy. We have to keep these fears and doubts to a minimum and replace them with helpful, exciting ideas of what we want our later life to be.

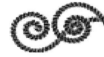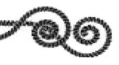

Here are a few examples:

- 70 is the new 40!
- As I get older, I have more choices than ever about how I live my life.
- The world is getting smaller . . . which means I can go places and do many more things than I ever could before.
- This world is filled with adventurous people just like me who want to live a juicy life!
- 90% of the things that people fear never come true. So all these fears about aging unhappily will not necessarily happen to me.
- I can be the total boss of the life I create.
- The #1 resource I need to live the life I want is creativity . . . and that is free!

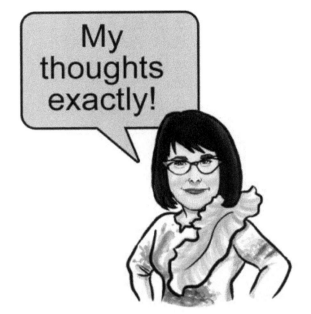

Just thinking happy thoughts is not enough. We have to be very deliberate in our actions, the kinds of people we associate with and the plans we make. It's been said that **"Failing to plan is planning to fail."** And as we plan for our later years, there is definite truth to this statement!

Despite society's expectations and your own fears and doubts, you must persevere. You are on a Quest!

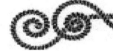
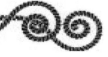

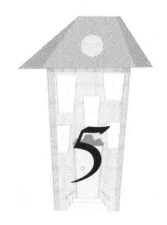

ONCE UPON A TIME

A Fairy Tale

*O*nce upon a time there was a woman named Gwendolyn who was growing more and more unhappy as she got older. Her village no longer felt like home and she longed for something more. Being the brave woman that she was, she set out on her Quest to find her home. She did not know where she was going or how she was going to find what she was looking for but she knew she must leave her village in search of a place that would give her true happiness.

For days she went from village to village searching for a place to call home. She would trek through forests and up and down mountains, but she found nothing that suited her. She began to feel very discouraged. One night while she sat by her fire eating her dinner, she began to cry. In her sobbing she looked to the sky and shouted, *"Why can't I find a place to call home? Somebody help me!"* Exhausted, she fell into a deep sleep. The next morning she awoke to continue on her journey. Walking through a forest glade, she came upon a large leather-bound book lying on the path. Picking it up, she found a note inside that read **"You can have what you want."**

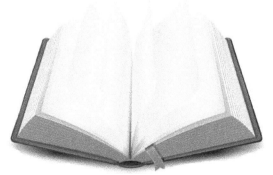

15

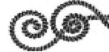
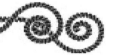

Befuddled yet excited, she flipped through the pages, but to her disappointment found every page blank. Her heart sank but she put the book in her bag and carried on down the path.

The next day, walking through a dark and somewhat eerie forest, Gwendolyn started to weep once more. When was she going to find her new home? How would she know where to go? At that moment she looked at the big Live Oak in front of her. Sticking out of the hole in the side of a trunk was a scroll. She removed the paper and saw the words **"Map to Somewhere"** *written on the front. Excitedly she opened the map and, like the book, found the page blank. She placed the map into her bag.*

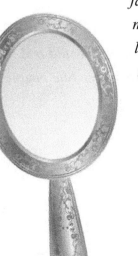

As she was looking for a place to set up camp for the night, she came across a young woman sitting on a rock crying. She went to the young girl to see what was the matter. The young girl's name was Phoebe. She told Gwendolyn she had been in the forest for weeks waiting for magic to happen and bring her the life she desired. Seeing that she was terribly upset, Gwendolyn invited her to stay the night with her, telling her she would help her find her way in the morning.

While the two ate their dinner, they talked about Phoebe's dilemma. She really didn't know what she wanted and she was afraid that she would never find happiness, never have the family that she longed for and would never have a place that would make her heart sing. Because Gwendolyn too knew what this felt like, she said to her, "Phoebe, I believe you can have a life that makes your heart sing. But it will not come to you, you will have to go and create it for yourself. But first you must believe it's possible. Then you must be brave enough to declare exactly what you think will make you happy . . . to ask for what you want. **Then you must start out on the path, even when you don't know where that path will take you.** *The young woman listened intently and soon both were fast asleep.*

The next morning when Gwendolyn woke, she found that Phoebe was gone. And in the place where she had slept was a mirror.

16

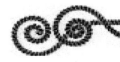
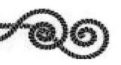

When she picked up the mirror and looked into the glass she heard words being whispered in her ear. **"Gwendolyn . . . you have everything you need. You know how to get it. Listen within and find your home."**

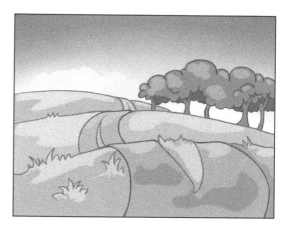

She pulled the empty book and the map out of her knapsack and laid them beside the mirror. "Were the answers here?", she wondered. But none of these things told her what to do. Out loud she exclaimed, **"I want to find my home. Where should I begin?"** *In that moment the book flew open and inside the words read, "***Take the first step and the rest will be made evident.***" In that moment the map opened and showed her a new path in the distance that awaited her. Excitedly she set off in the direction that the map told her to go.*

As she walked down the path, she came to a fork in the road. In truth, there were many ways that Gwendolyn could have gone. She consulted the map but the map did not give her the answer she needed. She held up the mirror and looking into her own reflection asked, **"Which way am I to go? What is the best way?"** *In that moment an arrow appeared on the map, pointing her in a new direction. Gwendolyn took that way, with a confidence in her step.*

Gwendolyn now had everything she needed to find her true place. She had information and answers to all her questions when she was courageous and wise enough to ask them, she had a map that would guide her along the many choices she would face, and she had a mirror which reminded her of her connection to others and the power of staying connected to her own true desires.

In a very short time Gwendolyn found the place that she would call home. It held everything that made her heart sing. And she lived HAPPY EVER AFTER.

THE END

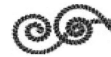
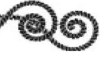

"Sticks in a bundle are
unbreakable."
Kenyan Proverb

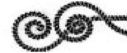
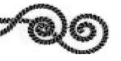

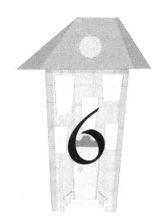

YOUR UNIQUE QUEST

Gwendolyn had the desire for a new way of living. But when she set out on her Quest she also held a few beliefs that weren't true. Those beliefs held her back.

First she believed that there was only one specific destination and all she had to do was find it. She also thought she could find it even though she didn't really know what she was looking for.

Secondly, Gwendolyn only began to feel and be successful when (in her frustration) she declared what she really wanted. Holding her dream lightly and without a lot of conviction and determination to find it, she remained lost. Only when she stated with confidence what she wanted was guidance revealed to her.

Information did not come to her in a clear succinct way; rather it often came in the form of **other questions.** Remember the book and the map? There was the potential for these to have answers, but instead at first they left Gwendolyn with more questions.

Isn't that how life is sometimes? The best thing we can do to find the answers we need is to be sure we are asking questions . . . and the right questions at that.

Then there was Phoebe. Alone Gwendolyn was at real risk for sinking into her own despair. She was finding it more and more difficult to continue on her search alone. But when she met Phoebe she found renewed energy. But perhaps most significant of all she found herself telling Phoebe the very things that she needed to hear herself. Isn't that amazing? We can

19

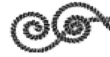
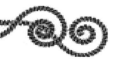

often see potential for others when we struggle to find it for ourselves. By championing Phoebe and her desire to have all that she wanted, Gwendolyn was renewed.

So, this Quest was not effortless. It was not simply "take to the road" and find exactly what you want. Gwendolyn's Quest was filled with walking down unknown paths, sitting in despair and having to pull herself out of the dumps. It required asking questions, the right questions, before answers could be revealed. Then and only then could she find the place, the home that she was looking for. Only after **making connections** to herself and others, **getting information** about a number of questions and **taking action** even when she was uncertain, could real progress be made.

In short, the keys to finding her real home were Connection, Information and Action.

"Whatever you can do or
dream you can, begin it.
Boldness has genius, power
and magic in it."

Goethe

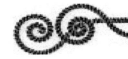
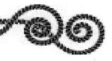

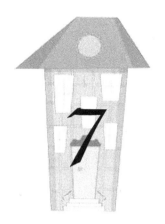

CONNECTION, INFORMATION AND ACTION

There are three essential ingredients to make your Quest successful.

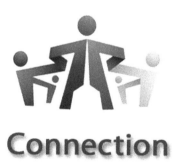

Connection

This is both an internal connection to yourself (your dreams, your desires, your strengths and your challenges) as well as a connection to people who are also on a Quest for Community. You will be asked to make connections all along this Quest. These connections will help us find many of the answers we are looking for. That's why it is one of the key ingredients in creating the Community you want, but also making and keeping that Community healthy.

21

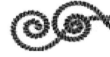
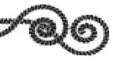

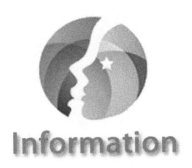

Information

What are you looking for? It's quite possible you don't know. To answer that question, you need information. Then once you make the decisions, there will be more information to gather. I recommend you start cataloguing this information by using this Guidebook, file folders or a notebook. But gather it you must. Information is the second key ingredient to creating the Community you want.

You can talk and talk and talk or you can research and research and research, but if you don't take action to make things happen you will never truly get to where you want to go.

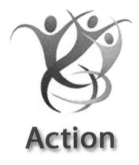

Action

Talking, planning, thinking and dreaming are important components of this Quest, but action is the key. Remember Phoebe and how she just waited for her Community to appear? She wanted it to magically manifest before her with little or no effort on her part. But it wasn't going to happen that way. It was never going to show up unless she took action. So, action is the third key ingredient of your merry Quest.

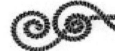
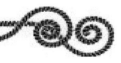

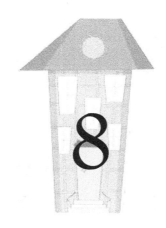

SELF-DISCOVERY

When I set out to intentionally find a Community in which to live, I had no idea I was also stepping into a profound opportunity to discover myself. I didn't know that in order to find people to live with – people I really WANTED to live with - I would have to know myself.

In truth, I thought I knew myself. I could have told anyone what I liked, what I didn't like, what my interests were, my fears, my joys. However, I discovered that some of those things I thought I knew about myself were now up for debate. Things were changing as I was getting older, deepening even.

So let me spell this out. If you want to live in Community, you will be discovering yourself, "the good, the bad and the ugly" as the saying goes.

On the following pages are a few questions/exercises to get you thinking about who you are and what you want.

NOTE: Don't write to impress. No one is going to read it but you, so putting a positive spin on everything won't help. Also, no one is going to judge you for writing down all your strengths, so go ahead and brag.

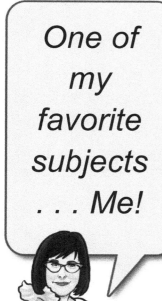

One of my favorite subjects . . . Me!

23

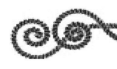
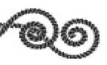

So, who are you?

Imagine you are applying for a job or signing up for an online dating service. You have to put who you are into words. Begin by answering the questions below.

Words to describe myself:

Career/Job History:

Partnerships/Romance:

24

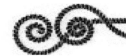
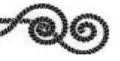

Children or Grandchildren:

My Values:

Education Level/Experience:

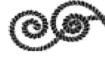

Finances/Economic Resources:

Faith:

Hobbies:

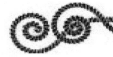
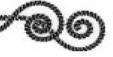

Favorite Books:

Favorite Movies:

Favorite Plays:

My Past Times:

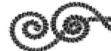

Marianne Kilkenny

Favorite Foods/Cuisine:

Places I like to hang out:

What I do for fun:

Political Views:

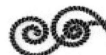
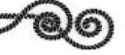

Exercise Habits:

Qualities I like about myself:

Qualities I don't like about myself:

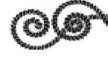
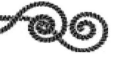

Friends tell me I am:

I'm excited about:

I'm afraid of:

Other things I want others to know about me:

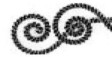
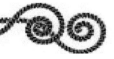

Taking the information from your answers to the previous questions, write a narrative that describes who you are. As you write it, imagine someone who does not know you will be reading it. Make it crystal-clear who you are. But don't overdo it. Just be honest.

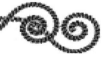

Digging Deeper

This is an exceptionally good start.   But let's be clear . . . the digging and unearthing and learning has only just begun. Just think about all the things you learned from living with others while you were growing up. That deep and challenging learning continues when you live in Community.

Zev Paiss, a fellow communitarian, has said living in Community is the **"longest, most expensive personal growth workshop you will ever be a part of."** I can promise you that deciding to form a Community and doing all the necessary steps to make it a reality will stretch you and make you grow.

"But that's a good thing, right?"

Yes . . . but lots of things that are good for us are not always easy in the moment.

"So what's so hard about it?" you may be asking.

1. You may see sides of yourself you do not like.

2. You may unearth memories or pieces of yourself that you wish had stayed buried.

3. You may feel vulnerable at times which makes you uncomfortable.

4. People may witness these parts of you and you may feel embarrassed.

5. You may try to create something and not have it turn out like you want it to.

6. You may feel fear . . . fear of rejection, of failure or of judgment.

7. You could actually be rejected, fail at this, or be judged.

8. You may fear that looking at the darker sides of yourself will open up Pandora's Box

    and unleash something that is too big or too hard to handle.

To name just a few . . .

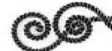
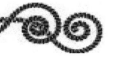

Are other challenges or possible blocks popping up? **If so, write them down here.** Simply getting them out of your head increases the chances they will NOT trip you up later. Like on a Quest, you have to prepare for a lot of different challenges and obstacles. Spending time before you leave preparing for Ogres and Dragons and Quicksand actually makes you less vulnerable if and when you meet them along the way.

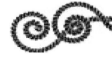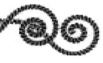

Now that you're awake and alert, let me tell you all the wonderful **benefits** you will receive as you allow yourself to dig deeper and get to know yourself as it relates to your Quest.

1. Like attracts like . . . so knowing who you are greatly increases your chances of attracting and being with others with whom you are compatible.

2. Knowing yourself is HONEST. And honesty is one of the core values and practices which brings people the freedom and joy they desire.

3. You can release parts of yourself that are old and stale and no longer useful. In other words, when you discover something you don't like about yourself, you are more likely to stop doing/thinking it!

4. Vulnerability is arguably one of the primary characteristics of a strong person.

5. You will be asked many times along this journey to share things about yourself. You will be prepared to have open, honest dialogue.

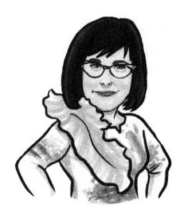

"If you are not willing to do this kind of personal reflection and to get to know yourself and to be vulnerable with others, living in Community may not be right for you."

Yes, I said it. So if your stomach knots up at the thought of doing this kind of self-assessment and sharing, perhaps now is not the right time.

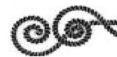
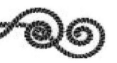

Your Values

Knowing your values is important, especially when you plan to live with others. Values are the attributes, virtues, actions and mindsets that are important to you. Values are something we all have; some remain constant throughout our lives and others change as we get older.

Below is a list of values one might strive to attain. It is definitely not a comprehensive list so I've given you some space to add to it. Rate each one below between 1 – 10 (with 10 being the highest) as to how important they are to you currently. ✳

_____Achievement

_____Adventure

_____Balance

_____Beauty

_____Community

_____Contribution

_____Family

_____Freedom

_____Friendship

_____Fun

_____Health

_____Justice

_____Love

_____Nature/Environment

_____Partnership

_____Peace

_____Power

_____Recognition

_____Self-Worth

_____Spirituality

_____Stability

_____Wealth

_____Wisdom

_____ _____

_____ _____

_____ _____

✳ *Adapted from material from the Center for Balanced Living*

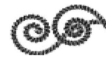
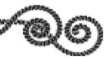

Listed next are values that could also be described as actions. In other words, the list below shows ways that one carries out core values. Do the same as you did with the other list. Rate each 1 – 10.

_____Accountability/Responsibility   _____Forgiveness

_____Affection   _____Honesty

_____Autonomy   _____Humor

_____Communication   _____Knowledge

_____Competency   _____Loyalty

_____Courtesy   _____Organization

_____Courage   _____Reason

_____Creativity   _____Safety

_____Discipline   _____Team

_____Drive   _____Tolerance

_____Fairness   _____ _____

_____Flexibility   _____ _____

_____Giving   _____ _____

What has this exercise revealed to you about yourself?

✱ *Adapted from material from the Center for Balanced Living*

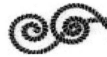
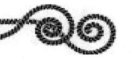

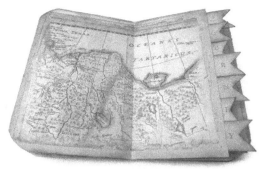

Travel Log

Use this space to organize information from the previous exercises, create to-do lists, and/or brainstorm the actions you want to take. Be sure to date your entries.

_____
_____
_____
_____
_____
_____
_____
_____
_____
_____
_____
_____
_____
_____
_____
_____
_____
_____
_____
_____
_____
_____
_____
_____
_____
_____

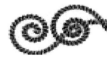
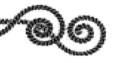

"The imagination equips us to perceive reality when it is not fully materialized."

Mary Caroline Richards

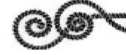
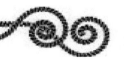

THE DRAGONS AND OGRES

No fairy tale would be complete without the evil "something" to fight—the Evil Queen, the Slobbering Ogre or the Fire-Breathing Dragon. So for you to start out on this journey and not expect to encounter any danger would be silly, now wouldn't it?

A worthy sojourner knows that danger could be around any corner so he or she needs to have his or her hand on the dagger, ready to fight to the death if necessary.

"What possibly could be so dangerous on my journey to find my Happily Ever After ?", you might be wondering. The dangers that lie before you, largely lie <u>within</u> you. Let me explain.

Steven Pressfield, in his book "Do The Work" writes:

> *"Our enemy is not lack of preparation; it's not the difficulty of the project or the state of the marketplace or the emptiness of our bank account. **THE ENEMY IS RESISTANCE.***
>
> *The enemy is our chattering brain which, if we give it so much as a nanosecond, will start producing excuses, alibis, transparent self-justifications and a million reasons why we can't/shouldn't/won't do what we know we need to do."*

There it is, our Dragons, the evil Ogres, the dark scary Monsters that threaten us. These evildoers can take many forms, but on the following pages are the most likely foes you will have to fight on your journey.

Let me introduce you to just a few . . .

39

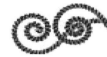
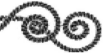

The Big Bad Wolf of Self-Doubt

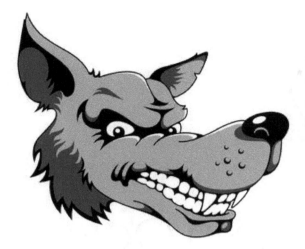

The Big Bad Wolf of Self-Doubt shows up a lot when we are undertaking something new. He comes along and whispers thoughts in our minds, telling us we can't really have or do what we want. He points out all the things that could go wrong or how we don't really have what it takes. Yes, the BBW of Self Doubt is a sly one. When he whispers these lies in our ears he makes us think that they are true. He can even conjure up circumstances the average person would see as evidence that "it" just can't be done. He loves it when we throw in the towel and give up.

Keep him out with
The Brick House of Faith

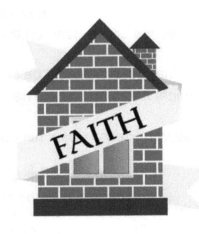

Doubts WILL come up along this journey, but the only real way to keep the wolf's fangs out of your hindquarters is to build a Brick House of Faith. Sharon Salzberg, in her book *Faith: Trusting Your Own Deepest Experience,* defines faith as "an absolute confidence in yourself." The Buddha says that "faith is the beginning of all good things." Building an internal foundation of faith, a belief in yourself and knowing that something great is just around the corner, will deter the Big Bad Wolf of Self Doubt.

How do you build this house? One brick at a time! Perhaps you hang **visuals** such as sticky notes or vision boards to remind you of what you want. Perhaps you have regular **connection** with others who have done what you want to do or are in the process of building Community. Perhaps you tap into the faith of your own spiritual practice and ask for guidance and support to keep the **faith**. Any and all of these can be the blocks of The Brick House of Faith.

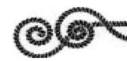
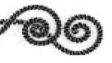

The Troll of Procrastination

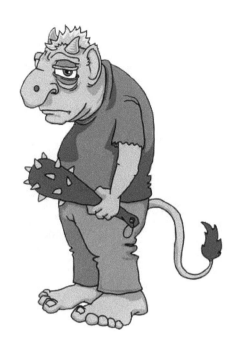

The Troll of Procrastination is a real bugger too. He is always getting in your way, especially when you are trying to get things done. You have to constantly step over him (or cross his bridge) in order to get where you want to go.

He is always there to point out there are other matters which need your attention. He insists that he will kindly let you cross his bridge AFTER you do those other things. He is masterful at holding you back.

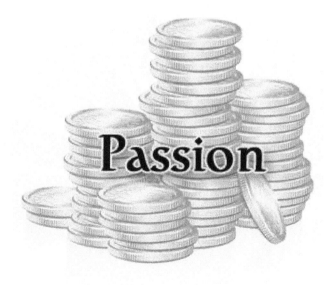

Pay him off with the
Currency of Passion

The Troll of Procrastination is no match for the Passion that you have in your heart for the things that you <u>really</u> want to do. In fact, it is this Passion that you can present to the Troll and he will let you pass. In other words . . . he can be bought off!

This Passion comes from within you—from identifying and then remembering what is really important to you. It is the root of self-discipline . . . remembering what you really want. There is a quote that says, "Don't let what you want <u>now</u> rob you of what you want <u>most</u>."

41

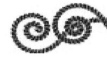
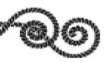

The Fire-Breathing Dragon of Distraction

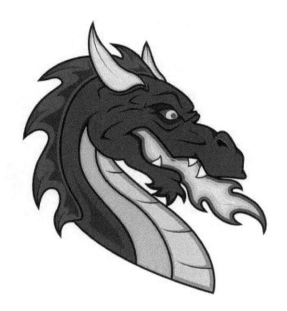

The Dragon of Distraction keeps you on your toes because you're never quite sure when or where she and her breath of flames will show up.

She draws your attention up and then down and then from side to side, keeping you constantly looking at what she wants you to think is most important. You feel that you have to put your attention where she is directing it because if you don't, you'll get burned.

Slay your distractions with the
Sword of Focus

The Dragon of Distraction is not as tough as she looks. In fact, in many cases she is just full of hot air. The best way to slay her is to wield the Sword of Focus.

This Dragon is simply no match for the power of crystal clear focus on what you truly want to have. The Sword of Focus takes some practice to use effectively. Clarity and focus can conquer distraction.

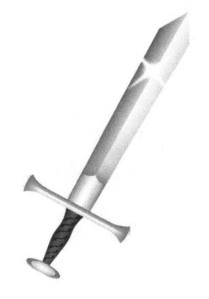

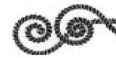

The Poison Apple of Perfectionism

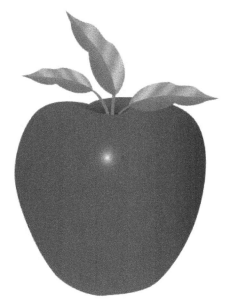

There's nothing like it . . . a flawless, shiny red apple without the littlest imperfection. But wait, is that true? Must an apple be perfect before it can be eaten and savored and provide nutrition? No, but this Poison Apple of Perfectionism will have you endlessly tilling and planting and pruning and nursing your project, convincing you that anything less than perfection is unacceptable.

Cure this with the

The Antidote of Good Enough

Don't let perfectionism get in the way of your success. Counteract that form of resistance with the Antidote of Good Enough. In truth, most often Perfectionism is a socially acceptable way of dealing with fear and self-doubt. But at its most basic, it's really resistance.

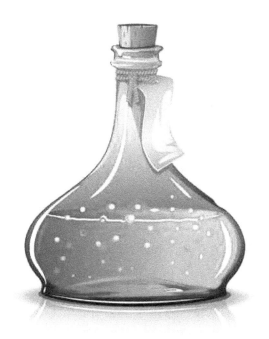

The Antidote of Good Enough helps you make peace with things when they are nearly perfect. The Chinese have a principle called Wabi Sabi which highlights the beauty of things that are imperfect, impermanent and incomplete. Nothing in nature is perfect—that is to say, without flaws. But everything is perfectly imperfect.

43

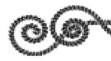
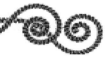

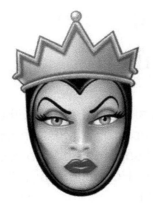

The Evil Queen of Fear

Fear is something we all feel, especially when we are doing something new. The Evil Queen of Fear knows this and does everything in her power to make you see and feel all the scary things associated with building your Community.

The Queen is quite beautiful and charming and can be very convincing. But underneath her beautiful and seemingly caring exterior is a desire to kill your dreams. We are afraid to get what we want. Ultimately we are afraid that we cannot ever have what we want. This greatly pleases the Evil Queen. "Fear saps passion."

Call upon your
White Knight of Truth

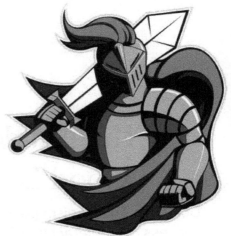

Fear can stop all of us in our tracks. It immobilizes our ability to see clearly and act on our own behalf. It distorts the truth, blows things out of proportion and is the ultimate creator of all forms of resistance. The thing that abolishes and dismantles fear is Truth. Ask yourself: What am I really capable of doing? What is the evidence that I can do this? What is the proof that I have that counteracts these beliefs?

The Queen knows that what you focus on becomes your reality. She will tell you that she is the fairest in the land and she is the only one that has your best interest at hand. But alas, she is lying. Your truth is your White Knight and it can set you free to follow the path to your dreams. The White Knight can overcome the Evil Queen of Fear by having you focus on what you want.

We often fear what we don't know. Or we take what we THINK we know and blow it out of proportion. Fear often seems to express itself in words such as "always" and "never." "I will never find people to live with." "I always seem to stumble when I talk about what I want." "No one will want to live with me." These are statements that simply are not true. The key to lessening fear is to be truthful with yourself. This means to accurately assess what is happening in the moment that is making you fearful. Let the White Knight of Truth come and set you free!

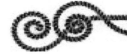
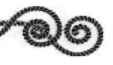

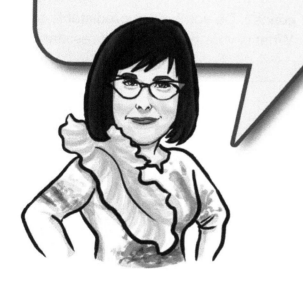

Here's the good news. Have you ever read a fairy tale where the dragon eats the princess? I haven't!

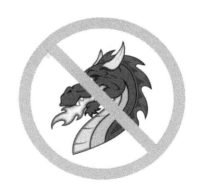

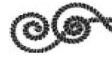

What will hold <u>you</u> back?

Okay, let's get personal. Think about a few times in your past when you wanted to do something different or new. Maybe you wanted to lose weight, or confront a friend about something challenging in your relationship. **What kept you from doing these things?**

Examples: Maybe you kept postponing your new diet and exercise regime. Perhaps you decided that you must have been wrong about the friend, so you didn't bring up your concern at all. List a few examples here.

Now take a look at your answers. What do you notice? Do you have a predictable pattern? Do you execute different resistance strategies? What is your typical form of resistance?

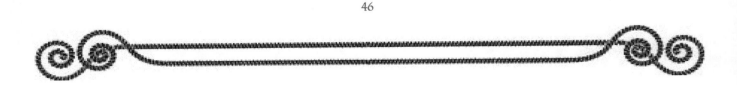

Next, take what you know about yourself so far and answer this next question.

What aspects or parts of your journey toward your Happily Ever After will likely meet resistance? And what will they look like?

Here are some possibilities to get you thinking:

- I won't have enough money.
- I don't know how much money it will take.
- It will take too much of my time.
- I don't trust that others will manage money as well as I do.
- I don't feel competent in financial situations.
- My life is too busy for this right now. I will do it later.
- I won't be able to find people who want what I want.
- This journey will involve a lot of meetings.
- What if I make the wrong decision?
- I will try too hard to please others.
- What if I change my mind?
- I will not get along with others.
- I will obsess over other people's annoying habits.
- I don't know what to do with all my stuff to downsize.
- What if hate it—how will I get myself out of it?
- What if I invest in this concept, hate it, and can't get out?

List some other possibilities below:

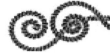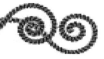

Now that you have identified the shape that your resistance might take, what is your plan? Will you build a Brick Wall of Faith? Fill your pockets with the Currency of Passion? Carry the Sword of Focus, keep the Antidote of Good Enough or call on the Knight of Truth? Or perhaps you have other strategies?

Some suggestions to help fight resistance:

- Find an accountability partner
- Hire a coach
- Make a vision board that will remind you why you want this
- Set time limits on research
- Set deadlines and put them on your calendar
- Look at your financial situation and know your real numbers

Write a statement or two or ideas about how you might fight when resistance comes up.

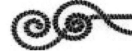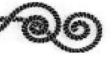

YOUR QUEST. . .IONS!

Below are the 5 tasks you will be asked to undertake along your Quest. Each one of these tasks asks fundamental questions. For example:

Personal Inquiry

What do I want? Where do I want to live? How much money do I have to put toward this?

Gathering Information

Who can answer my questions about the different geographic areas I'm considering? What kind of financing do I need? Who can I trust to give me the information I need?

Answering Questions

Can I rely on the information I get? How can I judge its quality? What do I do if and when I get conflicting information?

Deliberate Dreaming

Can I dare to imagine a life that really makes me sing? What does that look like? When do I stop dreaming and do something?

Taking Action

Where do I begin? Am I getting the results I want(ed)? What's next?

What do all these questions have in common? They are questions! Why, What, When, Where, Who and How—you will be asking yourself questions all along the process. But for simplicity's sake, I will take each of these "W" questions and break them down one by one.

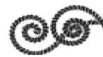
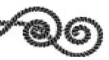

Map to
<u>Your</u> Happily Ever After!

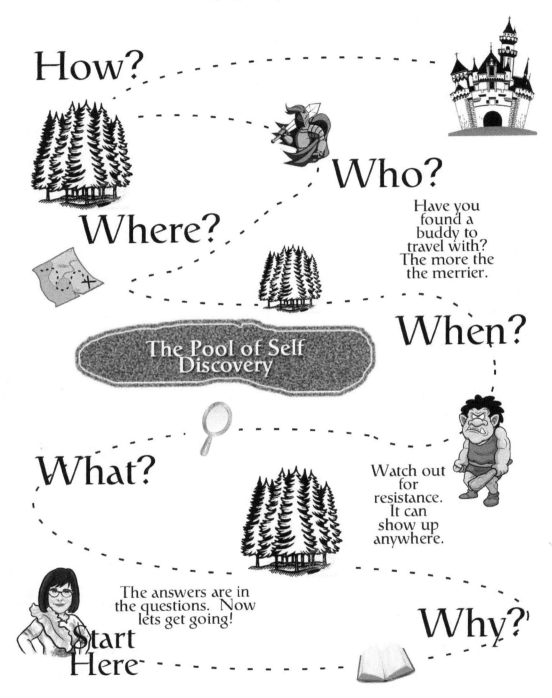

How?

Who?

Where?

Have you found a buddy to travel with? The more the the merrier.

The Pool of Self Discovery

When?

What?

Watch out for resistance. It can show up anywhere.

The answers are in the questions. Now lets get going!

Start Here

Why?

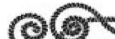
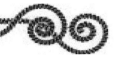

WHY?

WHY is quite possibly the most important question you will ask yourself . . . and one that is seldom asked. For this reason, we will begin here.

If you can't articulate **WHY** you want to live in Community, then you might not be able to get there. Asking (and answering) **WHY** allows you to get in touch with your motivation and what you would like the outcomes to be. Very often, without a genuine, internal connection to **WHY**, we often give up.

Let me give you an example. Let's say you want to shed a few pounds. You can define how much you want to lose, you can determine what you will do to make those pounds go away, and you can set deadlines and benchmarks and even ask for help from friends. But if you do you not have a compelling **WHY** that holds you to this goal, it will most likely fail.

Our **WHYs** are what really matter. Asking **WHY** you want something forces you to look at outcomes. Let's face it, there is a reason we want something and that reason must be clear.

Going back to losing weight, we could want to fit into a smaller size, we could want our triglycerides to decrease, and we could want to look better in a bathing suit. All of these are important and measurable. These outcomes could be enough to encourage us and keep us on a diet.

But what happens if we take it a little further and ask **WHY** again. **WHY** do you want to wear a smaller size? **WHY** do we want our triglycerides to be lower? **WHY** do we want to look better in a bathing suit? Get the picture? So enough about losing weight, let's talk about Community.

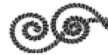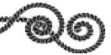

WHY do you want this? My guess is your answers will begin with the practical and the measurable. The answer might have things to do with companionship, finances, and support. That's all good. Begin there. But don't stop. Dig deeper. Keep asking yourself **WHY**, over and over and over.

Here are some questions to ask yourself with some possible answers:
Example #1:

> Q: **WHY** do you want to live in Community?
> A: My money at this stage will go farther if I live with and near other people.

> Q: **WHY** is this important to you?
> A: I have a lot of energy and a lot of years left. I want to remain active and have enough money to do all the things I want to do.

> Q: **WHY** is living a full life important?
> A: I've worked hard and postponed doing some of the adventures that have been calling me for years. I'm ready to fully explore other sides of me.

> Q: **WHY** is living an adventurous life important?
> A: I've watched friends and family shrink back from life and they seemed pretty miserable. Being happy is very important to me.

Example #2:

> Q: **WHY** do you want to live in Community?
> A: I don't have kids and I'm not married and the thought of living alone makes me feel sad and vulnerable.

> Q: **WHY** does living in Community sound appealing?
> A: I love being around people, helping them out and laughing. And I want to know that others are there for me. I thought that I would have that from marriage and kids, but that's not the case. I don't think I should give up on my dream just because I'm not in a relationship .

> Q: **WHY** does living in Community feel right for you?
> A: The short answer is I'm a people person and living alone no longer works for me.

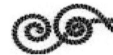
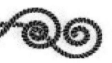

Do you see how this works? By asking **WHY**, you can get to the motivations of **WHY** you want something. You also get specifics that can be measured and you tap into the underlying feelings behind your desire.

So Now It's Your Turn

Here are the steps:

Step 1:   Brainstorm **WHY** you want to live in Community. Don't edit, just get the reasons down on paper.

Step 2:   Take each one of the entries on the brainstorm list and ask, "**WHY** is this important to me." Then write that down.

Step 3:   Go another round if you feel compelled.

Step 4:   Write your bullets and list as a narrative. Be sure to put the date on your entries. **This will be your foundation to come back to when things get rocky.**

Don't skip these next pages. They are very important!

On the following pages write your narrative in the form of a letter or email. Your task is to describe what you want and most importantly, **WHY** you want this. Remember, it's not about grammar and punctuation, it's about telling your story and tapping into the amazing power of **WHY**!

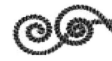
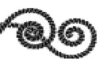

Step 1: Brainstorm why you want this.

This could be a bulleted list, a MindMap™ or just a page full of scribbles. Just get it down.

Step 2: Dig Deeper

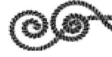
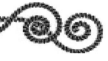

Step 3: Dig Even Deeper

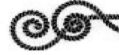
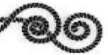

Write your "Compelling WHY" as a Narrative.

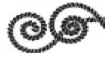

Marianne's Compelling WHY

September, 2013

My Situation:

I have lived alone for many years. I have no children, and I desire to live with my chosen family. Being divorced and without kids makes for aging that could be a lonely and difficult demise. I know I don't want to live in a conventional retirement home like my parents died in. That isn't for me. I want to live with others that I love and care about who really "know " me. That is my journey now. It has been for the last few years—finding the people, the place and how we get along together now based on information we have agreed on and continue to hone.

I choose to focus on polishing my rough edges off in a loving community of spirited individuals who take care of each other with joy and dignity. My contributions are received with generosity and aplomb.

My Vision:

Living in community allows for an easy and rich life in a safe and nurturing environment. Mutual support and spirituality are threads that run throughout all that we are and do.

We live in a village setting and the look is pretty, functional and assists us in human interaction with the allowance for privacy and alone time when we desire it. The layout follows principles of universal design, centralized common spaces and green principles, and movement away from automobile- centric living. Part of our community includes teaching and showing how it functions, the real-life stories and best practices in action. We offer classes, workshops and continuous learning about each other and making a connected world.

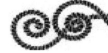
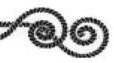

L. William's Compelling WHY

August, 2012

What is community? I live in a condo community. I have neighbors. Most I have never seen. Some exchange waves or smiles as we namelessly pass by. There are less than ten neighbors with whom I trade pleasantries or condo updates. In fact, if I didn't leave my unit for days, it would be quite a while before someone in this community came knocking on my door. Community to me is more than participating; it is sense of belonging in a group of people gathered together; it is a team spirit where we work toward the greater good.

In the second part of my life. I want to create my experience of living in a kindred spirit community by contributing my talent, time and treasure. I enjoy meeting new people, especially women who become part of my family, as chosen sisters. I value relationships. I feel a deep connection with other women. Within a few moments we can be laughing and exchanging points of view.

My energy is "Yes, I Can Do It!" I'm ready to step up. The time is ripe for discovery and seeing life in a new light. Traditional family units and financial protection steps are not security. I can meet my needs for loving relationships and combining resources by choosing to create and join a community. What would it look like?

Ask and it is given . . . So I am feeling the sense of wonder and satisfaction of having a loving diversified community of kindred spirits . . . in gratitude for living and sharing the human experience . . . traveling . . . learning . . . laughing . . .

I am beginning the process by making an intention to meet other explorers. So I have manifested an opportunity for me to learn from Marianne and meet curious and adventurous sisters who also want to explore varied models of women living in community.

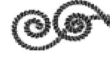
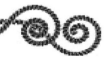

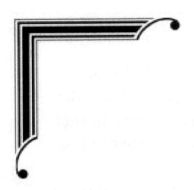

A Picture is Worth a Thousand Words

Instructions: Use these two blank pages to paste or draw images that represent your Compelling Why. You can also do this on a bulletin board or piece of poster board and then hang it in a place so you can see it every day.

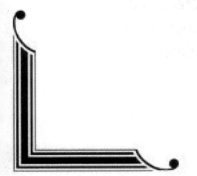

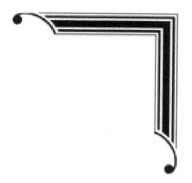

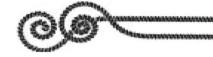

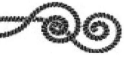

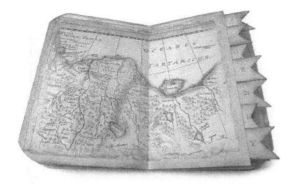

Travel Log

Use this space to organize information from the previous exercises, create to-do lists, and/or brainstorm the actions you want to take. Be sure to date your entries.

WHAT?

Getting to the Nuts and Bolts of Things

WHAT is another crucial question. **WHAT** do you want? **WHAT** does it look like, feel like?

This chapter is designed to help you describe and get clear on **WHAT** you want so you can go out and create/find it.

Let's begin with Community

Community is a dynamic whole that emerges when a group of people:

- participate in common practices

- depend upon one another

- make decisions together

- identify themselves as part of something larger than the sum of their individual relationships

- commit themselves for the long term to their own well-being, to each other, and to the group.

Adapted from "Creating Community Anywhere" By Carolyn Shaffer and Kristin Anundsen

63

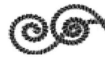
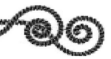

What exactly is out there anyway?

People living together and forming Intentional Community has always happened. Sometimes people have been thrown into a situation in which out of coincidence villages and towns were formed because people wanted to be in the same geographical locations. Many times people have selected their Community because they shared the same values, practices or desires.

Keep in mind, definition and terms are relative. You may meet someone who talks about cohousing yet is describing something completely different than the definitions given below. Always make sure you are referring to the same model when you are talking to others.

Intentional Community: "A group of people who have chosen to live together with a common purpose, working cooperatively to create a lifestyle that reflects their shared core values". *Federation of Intentional Communities*

Collaborative/Shared housing: A model of two or more unrelated people sharing a home. "It can be economical, sustainable, convenient and fun, and can offer many benefits." *The Sharing Solution*

Cohousing: A type of "intentional neighborhood" in which residents participate in the design and operation of the Community. Residents privately own their homes and do not pool their incomes, and there are common facilities for daily use. The decisions are made cooperatively.

Neighborhood/Villages: The focus is proximity to others for Community. They may be existing neighborhoods or a development of dwellings forming Community.

Concierge/Service: This is a model of services being brought to your home, wherever it may be. "Everything you need or wish you had . . . when you want it." *From Beacon Hill Village*

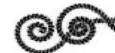
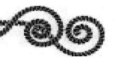

The Primary Variables of Community

There are at least 5 variables that when combined can make a plethora of Community alternatives.

- The Living Space

- The Location of the Living Space

- The Size of the Community

- The Composition of the Community

- Ownership and/or Finances

Living Space: This can range from what is currently called "tiny houses" of around 150 square feet up to any size you can imagine. Many people looking to live in Community are interested in downsizing and finding ways to live comfortably in smaller spaces. However this may not always be the case. Other aspects of determining the living space that is right for you is how much of the space is personal and how much is shared.

Location: Where is the Community geographically? Is it urban or rural? Near public transportation where driving is optional? Suburban? Is it self-contained with all of your necessities close by? Is it completely off the grid?

Size of Community: How big do you want your Community to be? Is it 2 or 3 people who want to live together in the same house? Is it a village-like development with 15 houses and a common house? Is it an apartment-like building with 30 or more residences? Is it a series of very small houses close by or one large house shared by many?

Composition of the Community: What is the composition of the people who live in this Community? Is it multigenerational? Is it age specific (50 plus years?) Is it for women only, men only, or couples?

Ownership: Do you own your own property and co-own some shared property? Are parts owned by all, and private ownership as well? Maybe you rent? Again, there are many different ways to configure ownership.

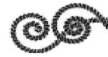
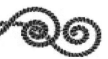

Okay, now what?

Begin by taking each of the 5 variables and doodle, brainstorm and journal about your current thinking on the matter. Make sure to date your entries. You might know exactly what you want, so write it down. On the other hand, you may have no real sense about what you want, but are very clear about things you do **not** want. Write that down too. Perhaps you can journal about different scenarios, asking yourself questions such as, "**WHAT** would I like about that?, **WHAT** would be challenging about that?, When I wake up each morning, **WHAT** do I want my ideal space to look like ? . . . how big is it? . . . do I have a cup of coffee or tea alone or with others?, How much space do I want and what do I want to share?"

Don't limit yourself to only those examples you've actually seen before, such as 5 people living in one house or a small neighborhood with single-resident bungalows. Visualize different combinations of the five variables. Branch out and consider lots of different possibilities.

So, dig a little. Connect within yourself and ask **WHAT** would be IDEAL for YOU! Play with these 5 variables and see what comes up.

Some Sample Configurations:

- Living in a large farm-like complex, sharing gardens and watching birds with other like-minded nature enthusiasts. We cook and share meals together several times a week but each of us has our own private living space. I rent my space and could leave at any time.

- An in-town urban apartment building within walking distance of most things I need. I share some time and space with other people who are the same gender as I am. Because we all like living in the city we dine out, attend plays and enjoy evening walks to people-watch.

- I own a nice big suburban home and rent out space to 3 or 4 people. Each day my path crosses with my housemates and we regularly share time together on the back porch. We throw parties together, go shopping and take care of one another's pets. We have established guidelines so everyone knows how to make this home run well.

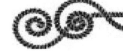
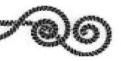

A Sample Configuration Matrix

Circle your desired choices, in each category, if you know what you want. This Matrix can be used to determine areas of similar and diverging interests and desires.

Living Space	Location	Community Size	Composition	Ownership
500 sq ft – studio	Urban Area (with no driving)	Village 12-15 units	Multigenerational	Rent
750 sq ft – 1 bd/bh or 1/1	Suburban – (close to services and must drive)	26 – 40 unit	Age specific 50 +_____ 55+ _____ Other ____	Buy
1000 sq ft 2/1 or 2/2	Self-contained complex (some services close)	4-plex or small configuration	Women only	Co-Ownership
1200 sq ft 2/2 or 3/2	Rural (must drive)	Large house to share	Men Only	Co-Rent
1500 sq ft 3/2	Off the grid	15 people	Couples	
House with 2 master suites				
Don't Know	Don't Know	Don't Know	Don't Know	Don't Know

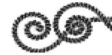
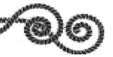

To Share or Not to Share . . . That is the Question

Living in Community is sharing and being with others. The more specific you can be about what you will and will not share, the better. You may not know exactly how you will feel until you actually live in Community, but I'm guessing you have some good ideas of what you want right now. Let's see.

Let's begin with a checklist. Put a "Y" beside the things which you would freely share. Then put an "N" beside those things you do not want to share . Put a "?" if you can imagine sharing them under certain conditions.

I wouldn't mind sharing my:

_____ House	_____ Yard work
_____ Car	_____ Housecleaning
_____ Kitchen	_____ Food
_____ Books	_____ Meals
_____ Bathroom	_____ Other _____
_____ Computer	_____ Other _____
_____ Yard tools	

Now transfer that list to the following table. Explain under what conditions you could or could not share.

Example:

Yes	No	Maybe
Meals	Food: I like to have my own, very specific groceries.	My Car: In an emergency, not on a regular basis
Kitchen	Computer	
Books	Bathroom	
Housecleaning		

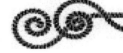
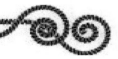

Now it is Your Turn

Yes	No	Maybe

Use the following pages to make notes, to doodle, to dream about the various things you want, don't want and aren't sure of. But most of all, remember . . . have fun!

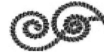
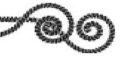

Living Space Desires

My "Must Have" or Deal Breakers

My "I Would Like to Have"

My "Not So Important"

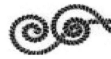
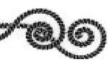

Living Space Notes

Make notes and jot down ideas about the kinds of living space you want.

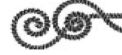
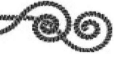

Location Notes

Make notes and jot down ideas about the location you want.

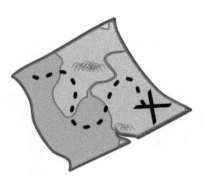

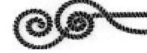 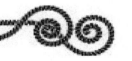

Community Size Notes

Make notes and jot down ideas about the size of Community you want.

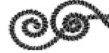
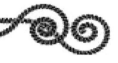

Marianne Kilkenny

Composition Notes
Make notes and jot down ideas about the kinds of people you want in your Community.

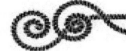
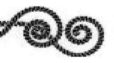

Ownership/Finance Notes

Make notes and jot down ideas about finances and ownership.

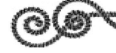
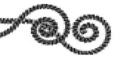

So . . . what do you want?

The clearer and more precise you are, the more likely it will be that you can find your Happily Ever After. You have to be able to describe it to others all along this journey so let's get it down and get it clear.

You've heard of the "elevator speech". It means being able to tell someone what you do for a living by the time the average elevator ride is over—let's say 60 seconds. But rather than describe our business we will describe what our Happily Ever After will look like.

And you already have all the pieces you need. In a sentence:

1. Describe your desired personal space (i.e. my own bungalow near others in a planned neighborhood, or a room in a large shared house)

2. How many people will you share this Community with?

3. Who will live with you? (All single women, shared spiritual practices, all retired golfers, etc.)

4. What do you want to share with others in your Community? (i.e. common living space, a kitchen, a car, chores, a garden, etc.)

Take from what you did above and plug in your answers to form your elevator speech. How does it sound?

> I am planning to live in Community. Ideally it will be made up of
>
> _____ and located in_____.
>
> My personal space would be a _____.
>
> All of the people who live in Community with me will share
>
> _____, _____ and _____.

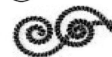
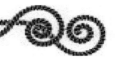

What are your Finances?

Obviously moving and/or creating a new place to live is going to involve finances. Determining what assets you have at the onset will greatly affect where you end up. It will also weigh heavily in the decisions you will make.

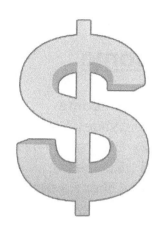

So what are your resources?

What do you have available to spend right now toward living in Community? What, if anything, will you be receiving at a later date? (For example, retirement, dividends, etc.) What are your expenses now and likely to be in the future?

These are important questions, so let's get the answers down on paper.

The following worksheets are going to ask you to look at your finances. You may be a person who already knows these numbers and for you, this will be a breeze. Or you could be the person whom knowing the "real numbers" is frightening or makes you anxious. If the latter is you, watch for resistance here.

Now is the time. Don't put it off! Get your head out of the sand and get your numbers on paper!

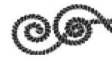

Delving into your finances is not a step you can skip on your Quest for your Happily Ever After. Well, you can, but it will keep rearing its head and holding you back if you don't take time to know and determine all you can about your financial situation. This truth telling will enable good and sound decisions in the future.

Make a cup of coffee or tea, maybe put on some music or light a candle and get busy. I can promise that doing this will make the rest of your Quest much easier.

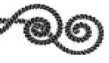

Marianne Kilkenny

Sample Monthly Budget Worksheet

Income

Earned income

1. Wages/Salary $_____
2. Bonus/Commission $_____
3. Business $_____
4. Other Earned $_____

Total Earned $_____

Unearned income

1. Retirement $_____
2. Pension and Profit sharing $_____
3. Social Security Benefits $_____
4. Alimony $_____
5. Interest $_____
6. Dividends $_____
7. Capital Gains $_____
8. Annuities $_____
9. Rent and Royalties $_____
10. Other _____
11. Other_____ $_____

Total Unearned $_____

TOTAL INCOME $_____

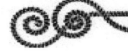
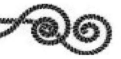

Expenses/Contributions

Fixed Expenses
1. Tithe $_____
2. Savings $_____
3. Emergency Fund $_____
4. Rent $_____
5. Mortgage $_____
6. Home Equity $_____
7. Home Improvement $_____
8. Automobile Loan $_____
9. Automobile Insurance $_____
10. Life Insurance $_____
11. Health insurance $_____
12. Disability Insurance $_____
13. Homeowners/Renters insurance $_____
14. Property taxes $_____
15. Cable/internet $_____
16. Other fixed expense $_____
17. Other _____ $_____
18. Other _____ $_____

    Total Fixed   **$_____**

Taxes
1. Federal Taxes $_____
2. State $_____
3. FICA $_____
4. Medicare $_____

    Total Taxes   **$_____**

Retirement
1. Retirement Contributions $_____
2. Other Retirement amounts $_____

    Total Retirement   **$_____**

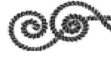
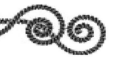

Marianne Kilkenny

Variable Expenses
1. Gas $_____
2. Electric $_____
3. Water/Sewer $_____
4. Telephone $_____
5. Maintenance $_____
6. Landscaping $_____

Total Variable $_____

Food
1. Groceries $_____
2. Restaurants $_____
3. Snacks/Take Out $_____

Total Food $_____

Auto
1. Registration/License $_____
2. Gas $_____
3. Oil/Repair $_____
4. Parking/Tolls $_____

Total Auto $_____

Miscellaneous
1. Bus/Taxi/Subway $_____
2. Childcare $_____
3. Clothing $_____
4. Medical/Dental $_____
5. Gifts $_____
6. Pet Care $_____
7. Other _____ $_____
8. Other _____ $_____

Total Miscellaneous $_____

TOTAL EXPENSES/CONTRIBUTIONS $_____

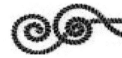
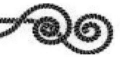

So now you have your numbers. Do your current finances support your vision? If not, what do you need? How far off are you now? What can you change? Do you think the numbers support what you want? Write about your thoughts AND your feelings about the numbers in the section below.

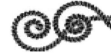
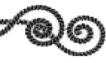

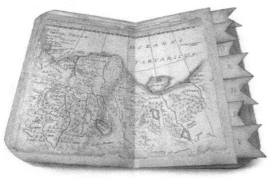

Travel Log

Use this space to organize information from the previous exercises, create to-do lists, and/or brainstorm the actions you want to take. Be sure to date your entries.

_____

_____

_____

_____

_____

_____

_____

_____

_____

_____

_____

_____

_____

_____

_____

_____

_____

_____

_____

_____

_____

_____

_____

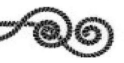

WHEN?

When Do You Want to Be in This New Community?

There are so many variables that affect this question and the answer depends on a lot of different things.

First, where are you in the process right now? If purchasing this Guidebook is one of the first things you've done, you may be quite a ways from moving into your Community. On the other hand, you may be someone who has been either consciously or unconsciously forming your ideas around Community for some time and there are only a few more steps for you to take. If that's you, then you might be moving into your Community soon.

Like many of the other sections, this section is filled with questions. These questions will help you determine what you want, what you know already, what information you have to seek out and what decisions you have to make.

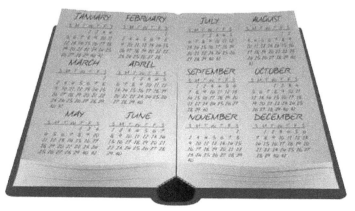

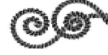
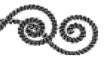

So let's begin talking about **WHEN**.

1. What, if anything, is happening in your future that would have a significant impact on your decision to form your Community? Brainstorm your answers below.

    Some examples might be: I'm retiring in June; I'm getting a divorce and need/want a new place to live; my daughter is having a child and she lives in Arizona and I want to move near her; my lease is up in 6 months.

2. Next, how soon do you want to make this a reality?

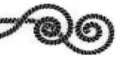

It's important to pick a date because it gives you something to work toward. **WHEN** a project is simply "sometime in the future" it is too easy to put things off, avoid answering some of the important questions and then taking action to get it done. In other words, we procrastinate. Yep . . . the Troll of Procrastination can rear his ugly head here and we have to conquer him by being clear and making ourselves set a date.

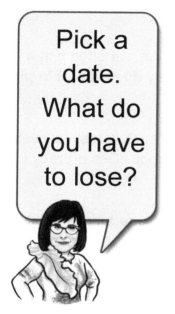

Pick a date. What do you have to lose?

But how do you do this WHEN there is not really an ideal time (except the fact that you're getting older)?

You just pick one. You simply think about it, look at a calendar and pick a date. It really doesn't matter **WHEN** it is but determining a goal date makes it real, keeps it a priority and taps into your internal sense of urgency.

You don't have to engrave it in stone. Things happen. Chances are once you get started, this date may change because of information you learn, people you meet, etc. But you still want to have a date—something that is firm enough to visualize and work toward but not so solid that you are unable to be flexible and go with the flow. It's that simple—or it's that complicated. Use your gut and your instinct and pick a date.

I will live in my Community

by _____.

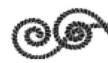
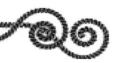

Finding your ideal Community is much more than finding a new place to live. This is a journey to CREATE the life you want. And during this Quest, you will discover things you need to learn, people you need to meet and lots and lots of questions that need answers.

Like Gwendolyn in our Fairy Tale, your next steps may not be explicit or clear. First you must ask the right questions, find specific information and learn what needs to be learned.

Using a Calendar

Calendars are one of the most basic time management tools we have. Yet, we often use a calendar only to schedule our day-to-day tasks and appointments. Rarely do we use it to **plan**. However, big projects require us to do just that.

First, determine **WHEN** you want the project to be done. Then, working backwards, we assign ourselves the various tasks that need to get done so we can reach our goal. This is pretty straightforward.

But what if there is not a predetermined completion date? **You must set one anyway.** Like I said before, without a target date we are all at risk of dragging our feet.

There is a reason you have me around. Come on!

On the next page is a simple example of how you could use a calendar. Once you've determined you goal date, plug in the other necessary tasks. I usually begin by making a master-list of all the things I need to do. Then working backwards, I place them on my calendar.

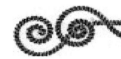
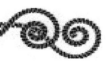

Example Calendar

January	February	March
• Complete the exercises in the Guidebook	• Coffee with Susan and Gerry • Look at cohousing Community across town	• Go to Meet Up
April	**May**	**June**
• Make a flyer about a potluck to talk about Community	• Host a potluck	• Have second meeting with interested people
July	**August**	**September**
October	**November**	**December**
January	**February**	**March**
April	**May**	**June**
		MOVE IN!

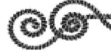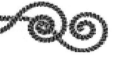

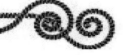

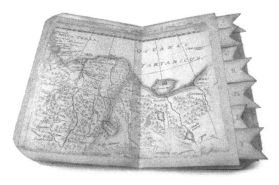

Travel Log

Use this space to organize information from the previous exercises, create to-do lists, and/or brainstorm the actions you want to take. Be sure to date your entries.

_____

_____

_____

_____

_____

_____

_____

_____

_____

_____

_____

_____

_____

_____

_____

_____

_____

_____

_____

_____

_____

_____

_____

_____

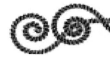 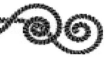

"You are never
too old to set
another goal or
to dream a new
dream."

Les Brown

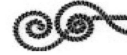
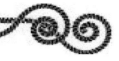

WHERE?

Location, Location, Location

WHERE do you want to live? Like the magical book that Gwendolyn found in our fairy tale, if you leaf through the pages of this Guidebook you will not find the answer to this question. There is simply no way for anyone else to know your heart's desire. But this Guidebook can help you uncover the answers.

Many of the questions you've already answered have gotten you thinking about **WHERE** you want to live. You may benefit from thumbing back through some of your previous answers to remind yourself what you have written.

If you already know **WHERE** you want to live, declare that right now! However, chances are you don't know and sifting through your options can be overwhelming. It's like going to a restaurant with a really large menu. Initially, we are delighted that we have so many wonderful choices. But then we find it difficult to narrow down what we really want. So let's break this question down a bit and look at it from a few different angles.

78% of you want to stay right where you are, not changing anything. Is this you? If it is, why are you reading this Guidebook? I bet some part of you wants to shake things up.

So keep re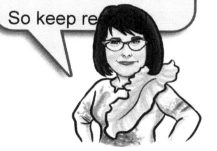

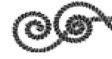
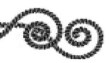

What do I want from the place where I live?

Read the list below and determine which of these items are important to you. Then rate them between 1 and 5, with 5 being of most importance.

_____ Quality public transportation	_____ Employment opportunities
_____ Driving distance to national/state parks	_____ Cleanliness
_____ Average temp of _____ degrees	_____ Near an airport
_____ Opportunities for continuing education	_____ City has a positive financial outlook
_____ University or college town	_____ Culturally and ethnically diverse
_____ Theater and the arts	_____ Politics are slanted toward your beliefs
_____ Active sustainability movement	_____ Active Chamber of Commerce
_____ Local symphony	_____ Active retirement Community
_____ Local sports team/s	_____ Beautiful architecture
_____ Vibrant downtown	_____ Historical roots
_____ High % of people in my age range	_____ Public gardens and green spaces
_____ Quality schools	_____ Affordability
_____ Clean water system	_____ Walkability
_____ Lots of quality restaurants	_____ Cosmopolitan feel
_____ Arts and crafts	_____ Laid-back easy feeling
_____ Live music	_____ Vibrant and bustling
_____ Bicycle friendly	_____ Street/music/art festivals
_____ Handicap accessible	_____ Proximity to water (lakes, beach, rivers)
_____ Access to quality healthcare	_____ Coffee houses & independent bookstores
_____ Weather is fairly constant	_____ _____
_____ Experience all 4 seasons of weather	_____ _____
_____ Access to a variety of shopping options	_____ _____

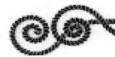
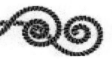

Use the space below to continue to brainstorm and prioritize the aspects that are most important to you.

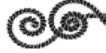

Next, transfer the information from the previous pages to the following categories using both what you know and your intuition.

Absolute Musts for Me	I Would Love It	Would Be a Nice Perk

If you are staying put, you may not need to do the following exercises in this chapter. If you are planning on relocating, I suggest you keep going.

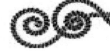
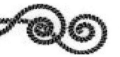

Which cities/places (that you know about right now) have many of the things that you want?

What research do you still need to do?
i.e. research on web, visit them, use your social networks.

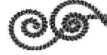
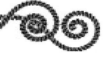

Are there people or places you want to be near? i.e. friends, grandchildren, the beach, the mountains, aging parent, etc.?

Do you want to stay in the US? If so, which areas call to you?

If not, what other countries would you like to consider?

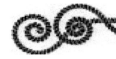

Digging Deeper About Your "Where"

You have research to do and some decisions to make if you currently don't live where you ultimately want to end up living.

1. Brainstorm possible locations that you are most interested in.

2. Now put this list in order of your preference.

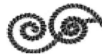
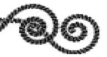

3. Put each location on a separate sheet of paper.

4. Make a list of your questions associated with each city or place. Then, go out and find the answers. How, you might ask? Here are a few ideas to get you started.

    a. Begin with the Internet. Most cities have a website through their Chamber of Commerce. Begin there.

    b. Read an article written about the city you are interested in.

    c. Do you know someone who lives there? If so, pick up the phone and call them.

    d. Use social media. For example, post a question on Facebook™:"I'm considering moving to Austin, Texas. I would love to chat with folks who live there. Please let me know if you would make time for a conversation."

    e. Take a trip there to look around. Obviously you will want to visit the city you ultimately choose, but what about scheduling a little vacation get-away? No research can compare to hands-on, drive-around-and-get–a-feel-for-the-place experience.

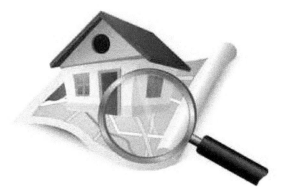

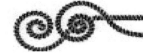
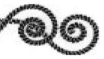

I'm considering _____

(City name)

Steps I need to take:

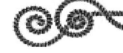
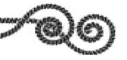

I'm considering _____

(City name)

Steps I need to take:

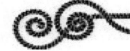
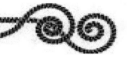

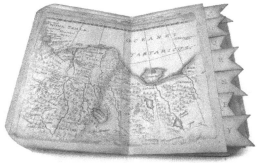

Travel Log

Use this space to organize information from the previous exercises, create to-do lists, and/or brainstorm the actions you want to take. Be sure to date your entries.

_____
_____
_____
_____
_____
_____
_____
_____
_____
_____
_____
_____
_____
_____
_____
_____
_____
_____
_____
_____
_____
_____
_____
_____
_____
_____
_____

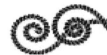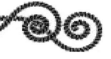

"If you knew who
walks beside you
on this path that
you have chosen,
fear would be
impossible."
                    Course in Miracles

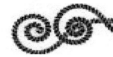
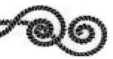

WHO?

I imagine this question feels like both the most important and the scariest to consider. "Will I really find people who will all get along, want the same things, and respect one another?"

Yes, you will. But it doesn't happen by accident.

As we look at the question of "**WHO**", there are really two different questions.

The first question is **"WHO do I want to live with?"**

Other questions that are connected to this primary question are:

- **WHO** do I NOT want to live with?
- **WHO** are the people who are already interested in living in Community?
- What kinds of personality types would be easiest for you to live with? The most challenging?

The second "**WHO**" question is **"WHO can help me find them?"**

Just like in previous chapters, we have to ask more questions.

Let's begin by going back to page 31 and rereading the narrative you wrote about yourself.

Now that you've refreshed your memory about what you wrote earlier, let's dig some more!

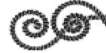
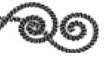

WHO do you want to live with? Do you already have actual people in mind? If so, write their names down here and why they are a fit for you.

Ideal Characteristics of People In My Community

Below are traits of people you might want to live with. Using the list below, determine which of these characteristics are important to you. Then rate them between 1 and 5, with 5 being the most important.

_____ is a woman

_____ is a man

_____ is either a man or woman

_____ has the same sexual orientation as me

_____ has similar financial resources as I do

_____ is exceptionally neat

_____ is moderately neat

_____ shares my passion for_____

_____ likes dogs

_____ likes cats

_____ does not have any pets

_____ shares my same political views

_____ enjoys a healthy debate about ideology

_____ is religious and/or has a strong faith

_____ has religious beliefs that are similar to mine

_____ is physically fit and healthy

_____ is a vegetarian

_____ is an avid reader

_____ likes to garden

_____ is talkative

_____ is quiet and reserved

_____ practices healthy communication

_____ is responsible with money

_____ is a good sharer

_____ is respectful of other's boundaries

_____ is decisive

_____ is thoughtful about making decisions

_____ is a risk taker

_____ is cautious in most areas of his/her life

_____ values time with family

_____ likes to play golf

_____ likes to play tennis

_____ likes to play racquetball

_____ likes to hike

_____ likes to go fishing

_____ likes to visit museums

_____ likes to go to art galleries and openings

_____ likes to go to live theater

_____ likes to go to the movies

_____ likes go out to eat

_____ likes to host parties

_____ likes to celebrate mainstream holidays

_____ would consider him/herself liberal

_____ would consider him/herself conservative

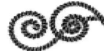
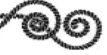

Use the space below to brainstorm and prioritize additional characteristics/aspects that are most important to you.

Next, transfer the information from the previous pages to the following categories using both your knowledge and your intuition.

Absolute Musts for Me	I Would Love It	Would Be a Nice Perk

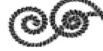
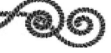

Marianne Kilkenny

So, you've got some idea of the kinds of people you want to live with. Let me guess what you are thinking. . .

"Where are they?"

They are out there. But you have to use your connections, seek out some information and most importantly take some deliberate, thoughtful action to find them.

To do this, I'm going to walk you through creating a social MindMap™ of sorts for this purpose.

For our purposes we are going to build a MindMap™ around who you know and who they may know. A mind map is a diagram used to visually outline information. You can find out more about Mindmaps™ online.

You will begin by thinking of people with whom you interact personally such as co-workers, colleagues, family, friends, etc. Then you go on to identify who they may know.

Here are some suggestions to get you going.

<u>Family members:</u> Parents, siblings, aunts, uncles, cousins, long-lost cousins twice removed, your in-laws and their families, etc.

<u>Friends:</u> Your best friends and your immediate circle of friends, your neighbors, people with whom you go out to dinner or lunch (look through your calendar to jog your memory), people on your holiday card list, etc.

<u>Colleagues:</u> People you work with now or have in the past, people whose line of work intersects with yours, past clients or customers, etc.

<u>Organizational Connections:</u> People you know from church, synagogue or mosques (current and past participations), sports teams or fans, high school friends, college friends, professional association members, book groups, support groups, club members, special interest groups, political friends, etc.

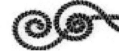
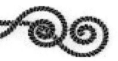

Step 1: Draw a circle in the center of a page and place your name in its center.

Step 2: Then draw a line from the center circle leading to another circle in which you will place the name of an individual you directly and regularly connect with.

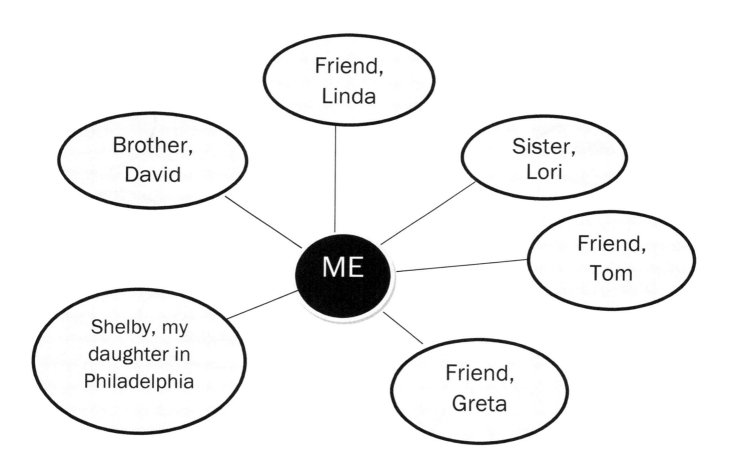

Step 3: Then think about acquaintances and groups that you are part of. Make a circle for each of those and draw a line to the center circle.

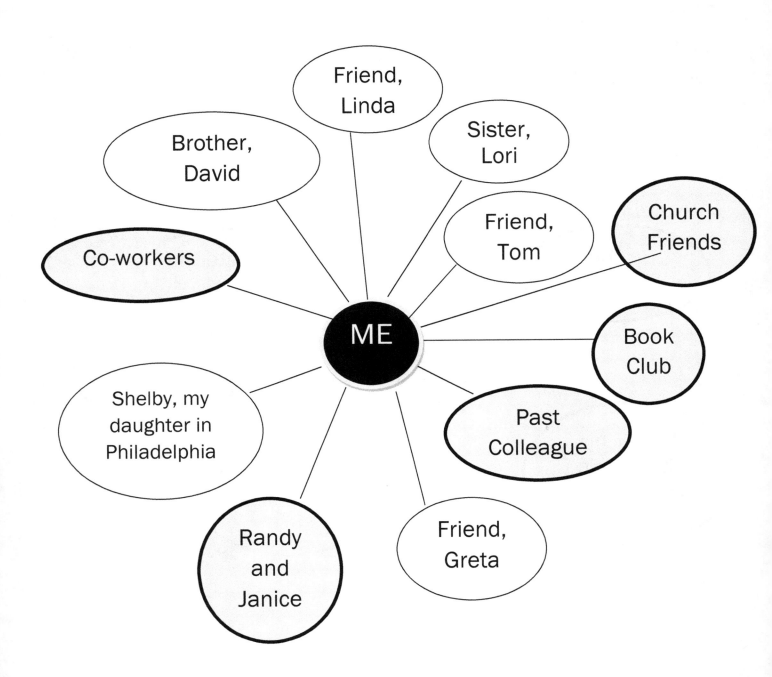

Step 4: Take it as far as you want to go!

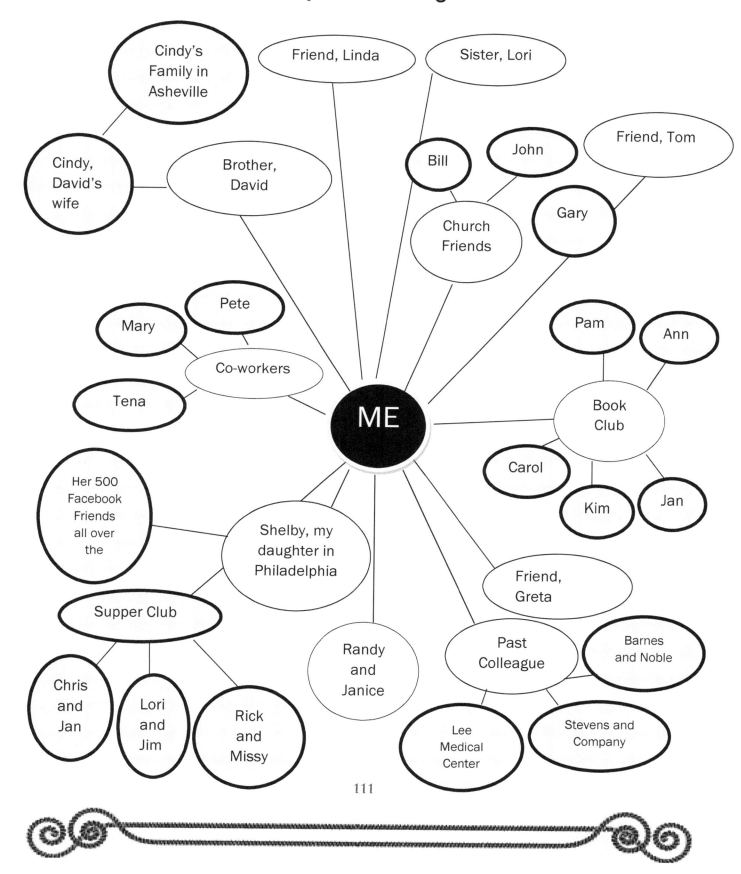

Here is a blank page to get started. Get a larger piece of paper and maybe even some colored markers or pencils and GO TO TOWN! You will be amazed at just how many connections you have.

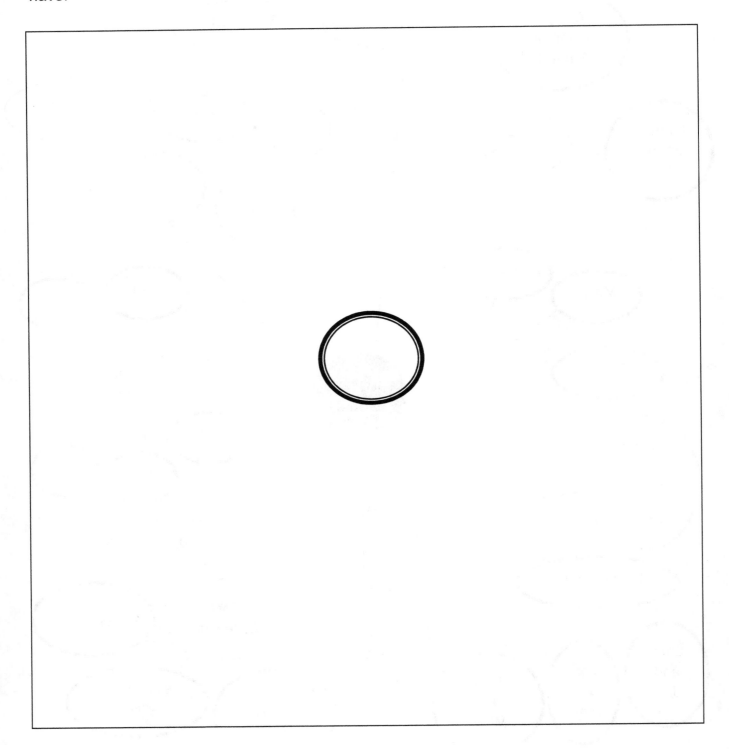

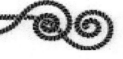

Honoring "No"

By now you are getting a picture of the types of people you want to live with—on paper at least. But that may not be enough.

Your intuition (or gut feeling) plays a vital role too.

Listening to your intuition may sound simple, but surprisingly many of us don't do it. We ignore our internal red flags. Our desire for Community could be so great that it overpowers our intuition, making us blind to the warning signs that someone is not right for us.

The good news is that this nagging feeling can be equally as persistent and will continue to send us signals that require our consideration. Our job is to pay attention. So, when you get a red flag that someone is not right for you, listen . . . then say "No".

You have an inherent right to your opinion. Own it and use it!

113

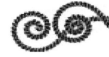
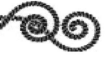

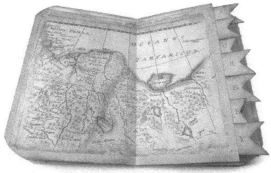

Travel Log

Use this space to organize information from the previous exercises, create to-do lists, and/or brainstorm the actions you want to take. Be sure to date your entries.

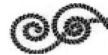
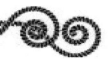

HOW?

HOW is the sixth and final question.

I have chosen to address **HOW** last. Many people begin with **HOW** because they find it the easiest and most concrete place to begin. However, I hope you will see the importance of beginning with the other questions first.

When you have the answers to Why, What, Where, When and Who, then **HOW** becomes quite easy.

I've heard it said that "**HOW** is none of your business." This used to confuse me. "**HOW** can **HOW** be none of my business?" I've come to understand that this statement means we need only to simply take action toward what we want and the specifics will work themselves out.

- "**HOW** do I find people I want to live with?" You begin by talking to others about your vision and then people will begin to show up.
- "**HOW** will I know where I want to live?" You can poke around on the Internet or go on weekend trips to places you are considering. These activities will help you get clearer about the kind of place you want to live.

What I've described is called serendipity. Serendipity is "the occurrence and development of events by chance in a happy or beneficial way". When you start setting goals and making plans, the things, people, and opportunities you need will begin to appear.

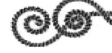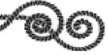

Some HOW Questions to Consider

There are many **HOW** questions which need your attention. Below are a few for you to ponder. Finding the answers to these questions will ultimately help you on your Quest. So let's get digging again!

Below are some of the questions which you have already addressed in the previous chapters. However, take a bit of time and jot down the answers once again. It will help you refine your ideas even more and highlight where you need to do some more work.

HOW will I decide where I want to live?

HOW will I know when something is a good fit?

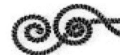
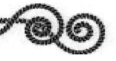

HOW will I know when something is a mistake?

HOW will I stay focused and not give up or get discouraged?

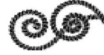

HOW much money do I have available to put toward this project?

HOW do I make important decisions?

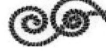
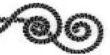

When conflicts arise, **HOW** do I want to handle them and myself?

"**HOW**" is a one-step-at-a-time kind of thing. It is pulling together lots of information and then finding a way to take action. Here are a few tips:

1. Be as clear as possible about what you want

2. Be equally clear about what you do **not** want

3. Set specific goals

4. Set measurable outcomes that you want to create

5. Use your calendar as a tracking tool

6. Watch for and deal with resistance

7. Revisit some of the earlier parts of this Guidebook often

8. Take a break

9. Find others who are also on this Quest and travel together

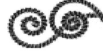
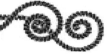

Characteristics of a Successful Seeker

A Depth of Knowledge
Success seekers have a desire to know and they seek out the answers. They are not stumped by the questions; in fact they ask more so they can go out and find the answers.

Introspective
They go deep inside themselves to understand themselves as best they can. They take time to look inside at their fears, their strengths and their motives.

Risk Takers
They don't let a little fear or a little challenge knock them off balance. They face their challenges head on!

Natural Yearning for Connection with Others
They genuinely like people and value what it means to be in Community. They don't have to be with people all the time, but they have a natural desire to belong.

Willingness to Sacrifice
They understand that sometimes they have to let go of something in order to get something else. They appreciate that sacrifice is often a part of any journey that is worth taking.

Flexibility
They are not rigid and set in their ways. While they know what they want and think positively about getting what they desire, they remain flexible to what the circumstances require of them.

Willingness
They are enthusiastically willing to go after their dreams.

Sense of Adventure
They have a twinkle in their eye as they look for new and exciting opportunities to grow and learn. They don't let a little fear keep them down.

Open to Grace and Magic
They actually expect that the world will open up to them and opportunities will arise.

Now reread the list of characteristics and think of Gwendolyn, our Seeker who set out on her Quest to find her Happily Ever After. Which of these characteristics did she possess before she left? Which ones did she gain along the way? Which of these do you have? Which of these do you want to develop?

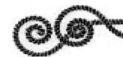
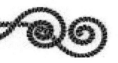

Which of these qualities do you currently possess?

Which ones are you missing?

Which ones would you like to develop in yourself?

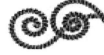
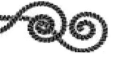

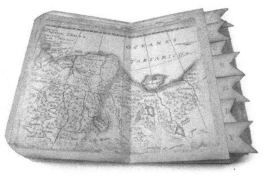

Travel Log

Use this space to organize information from the previous exercises, create to-do lists, and/or brainstorm the actions you want to take. Be sure to date your entries.

_____
_____
_____
_____
_____
_____
_____
_____
_____
_____
_____
_____
_____
_____
_____
_____
_____
_____
_____
_____
_____
_____
_____
_____
_____

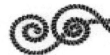
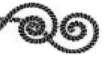

How?

___ Complete "How" Questions to Consider
pg 116-119

___ Complete
"Are You A
Successful Seeker?"
pg 121

___ Complete
"Absolute Musts"
pg 107

___ Complete
"Ideal Characteristics
of People"
pg 105

___ Complete
"Who You Know
Mindmap"
pg 112

Who?

___ Complete
"Location
Determination"
pg 96-98

___ Complete
"What Do I Want"
Checklist
pg 92

Where?

___ Complete
"Absolute Yes List"
pg 94

___ Declare a Target
Move Date
pg 85

The Pool of Self
Discovery

When?

___ Complete
"Financial
Worksheets"
pg 78-81

___ Work with the
Configuration
Matrix
pg 67

___ Complete
"Living Space
Desires"
pg 70

___ Complete
"Elevator Speech
about What you
Want"
pg 76

___ Complete
"To Share Or Not
To Share?"
pg 68-69

What?

___ Gather Pictures
of Your Vision
pg 60-61

___ Write Your
"Compelling Why"
pg 57

___ Brainstorm
"Why You Want
Community"
pg 54

Why?

Your
Journey
Begins

___ Sign
Committment Sheet
pg 11

___ Complete
"Who Are You?"
pg 24

___ Complete
"What Will Hold
You Back?"
pg 46-48

___ Gather your
Knapsack items

___ Complete
"Your Values"
pg 35-36

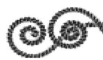
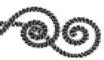

On the preceding page is a map of your Quest. Use it to keep track of what you have done.
Put a check beside the tasks or exercises as you complete them.

How can you celebrate your progress and/or accomplishments?

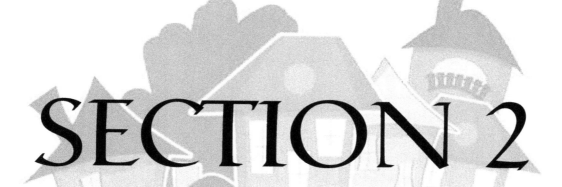

SECTION 2

FINDING TRAVELING COMPANIONS
(YOUR BAND OF MERRY MEN AND WOMEN)

"I jumped off
the cliff, and
everything started
falling into place."
Karina Gentinetta

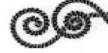
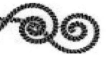

Finding Your Community

The goal is to live with others, right? But how do you put people from all different walks of life, with different values, of different ages, and different genders together in this environment you are creating?

VERY CAREFULLY!

To form Community right, you must be intentional. Not only do you have to seek out people who are interested in living in Community in the same way you do, but you also have to be compatible.

Compatibility means the ability to live in harmony. Let's face it; living in Community you are going to have to take deliberate steps to make it harmonious. Some of the tools in this section are to help facilitate that harmony—from getting to know one another at the beginning of the journey to dealing with issues later as they arise.

First of all, where are these people? In truth, they could be anywhere and everywhere. They could be people you already know, friends of friends, or complete strangers. No one wears a sign that designates them as someone interested in living in Community so a special effort has to be made to find one another.

127

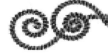
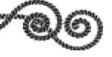

But no fear . . . like-minded people find each other all the time. They do so by:

1. making it known what kind of people they want to be with

2. going where those people are

3. creating an opportunity for people to self-identify and then come together

For Example:
People interested in politics or cultivating a certain hobby might volunteer for a campaign or take a class. People interested in fitness might join a gym where they find other people with a similar interest.

The web provides countless opportunities for like-minded people to find one another in chat rooms, web-based communities and even facilitating face-to-face interactions. Two examples are Match.com™ for people who want to make themselves available for dating and MeetUp.com™ for people who want to start a specific group or find a group around a particular topic or interest. There are countless others, but suffice it to say, it has never been easier to find specific kinds of people.

But that is not to say it is easy. It can FEEL like trying to find a needle in a haystack.

1. You begin by finding the people who have living in Community on their mind, or if exposed to the idea, would be game to explore it.

2. Once you find those people, you begin conversations to determine if what they are looking for is similar to what you are looking for. Do these people want the same kind of place and setting as you? Do they have similar resources and timing concerns?

3. Then you continue to work further to find more people with things in common with you, until eventually you have critical mass (a number that will depend on what you are trying to create) and are ready to start building your Community.

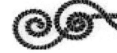
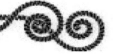

The Whole World

People who are thinking about how to live out their later years

People who are interested in the idea of living in community

People who are ready to form a community

People who know what they want in a community

People who want what I want!

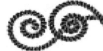

Marianne Kilkenny

PITFALLS AND OTHER TRAVESTIES

WHAT COULD GO WRONG?

Because I believe in this process, and have faith you can find Community, I warn you about the negative things that can happen. You are beginning a journey to find your Happily Ever After. Have you ever known a hero or heroine who did not run into some kind of trouble along the way? Here are a few pointers about the scary things you could encounter so you will be prepared to deal with them or avoid them entirely.

Holding onto the Past: "This is not how it should be." "This is not the way I've done it in the past." Everyone in your group will come with a lifetime of experiences. These experiences influence the future. As the saying goes, an unexamined past is destined to repeat itself. Having said that, this is a new adventure you are on—one in which many of the ideas you will be exploring will fly in the face of the way you thought they would be. In this case, it is best to let go of the way things used to be and embrace the new.

Fault Finding: When things aren't going the way we want them to, it is very easy to place blame. You may blame others or blame yourself. Either way, spending energy trying to determine who is responsible for things going wrong is a waste of time—time that is far better spent looking for ways to make things work.

A Lack of Shared Understandings: Much of this journey involves being with other people—people who have different experiences, ideas, desires and ways of doing things. Trouble is just around the corner if you and whoever you are working with do not have a predetermined way of dealing with each other and different scenarios. For example, you need to determine BEFORE IT HAPPENS, what you do when you disagree. How do you make decisions? Not having agreed-upon understandings and a decision-making process is a recipe for disaster.

Triangulation: From Wikipedia, "The term triangulation is most commonly used to express a situation in which one family member will not communicate directly with another family member, but will communicate with a third family member, which can lead to the third family member becoming part of the triangle." As the definition describes, it originated in a study about dysfunctional families. But as you can imagine, this can occur in other communities as well.

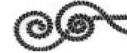
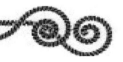

Horror stories: You won't have to look far to find someone who has a cousin who had a friend who tried to live in a shared house and it didn't work out. Why are people always so eager to share stories of when things didn't go well? My guess is they are trying to be helpful, but in truth it really isn't. So when someone starts to tell you a cautionary tale, kindly tell them thanks, but keep it to themselves.

Lack of communication & communication skills: Both Community and communication come from the Latin word *communicare* which means to impart, share and make common. So the keystone to a solid Community is good, quality communication. This means a lot of things. Talking to one another, being clear, agreeing how you want to communicate, having rules about kindness, use of tools like Non-Violent Communication and The Blueprint of We that have been tested. (See Resources on page 175) The lack of communication or when it is done poorly is the number one reason communities don't work. Communities are simply a web of relationships living in proximity.

No exit strategy: Before you really get started forming a Community with others, you have to assume that at some point someone may change their mind and/or want to leave. If you wait until this happens to decide how it should be done, you are asking for trouble. Take the time on the front end to decide how someone may leave if they choose.

People don't know themselves: It is my contention that individual must know themselves well in order to form a solid Community with others. But not everyone knows this, especially when they start out. So it's no wonder that trouble can come up. Knowing yourself doesn't prevent problems but it sure makes them easier to navigate.

Halo Effect: Have you ever been in a situation where you wanted to believe it was far better than it really was? Maybe it was someone you dated. You liked certain things about them so much

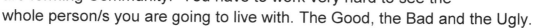

I recommend that when you find people you want to form Community with, that you ask them to get this Guidebook and do some digging themselves. Might save you lot of headaches in the future.

you were blind to some negative attributes. This is called the Halo Effect. Just like in dating, this can also happen when you are forming Community. You have to work very hard to see the whole person/s you are going to live with. The Good, the Bad and the Ugly.

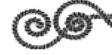
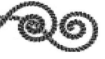

And Another Way to Look At Things

Here's a graphic representation of the steps you take to find and cultivate your Community. Don't let the arrows confuse you. You may go forward, backward and forward again many times to find your Happily Ever After.

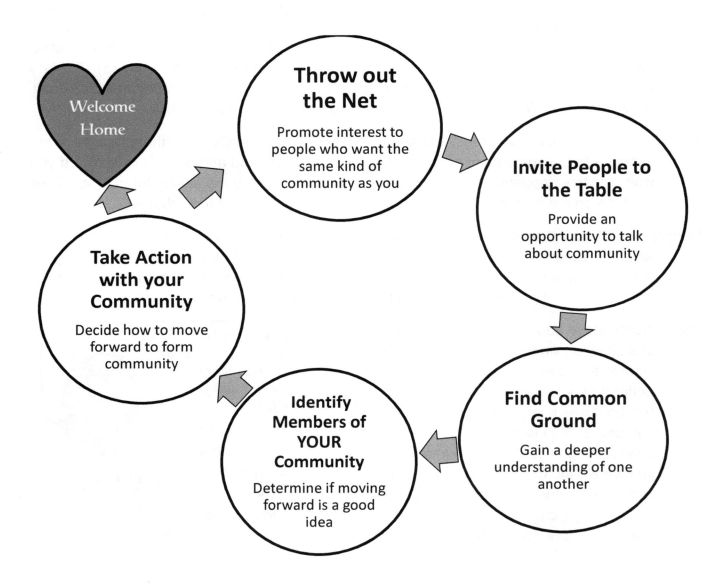

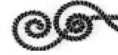
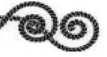

Travel Log

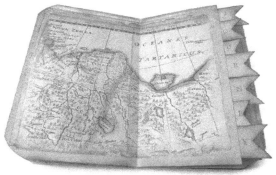

Use this space to organize information from the previous exercises, create to-do lists, and/or brainstorm the actions you want to take. Be sure to date your entries.

_____

_____

_____

_____

_____

_____

_____

_____

_____

_____

_____

_____

_____

_____

_____

_____

_____

_____

_____

_____

_____

_____

_____

_____

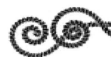 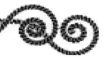

"For millions of years, human beings have been part of one tribe or another. A group needs only two things to be a tribe: a shared interest and a way to communicate."
Seth Godin

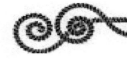
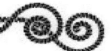

THROW OUT THE NET

PROMOTING INTEREST IN LIVING IN COMMUNITY

Now your task is to find the people you could potentially live with. How do you do this? Ironically, the same way you might find a new baby sitter or lawn service. **You ask around.**

You need to let it be known (or advertise) that you are trying to form a Community and want to attract others who might be interested too. To do this, you have to get the word out. There are many ways to do this, but here are three ways that I have found to be the most successful:

- Face-to-Face Conversations
- Social Media
- Placing Advertisements

Face-to Face-Conversations

Begin by stirring up interest. Or at the very least you have to tell your network what you are trying to do so you can find other like-minded people. It is hard to comprehend how many people we are connected to. Not only are we directly connected to many people, but those individuals have their own networks as well that we are indirectly connected to. If you did the exercises in Chapter 15, you already know your network of people and who you are directly and indirectly connected to is much larger than you may have initially thought.

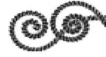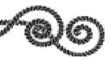

In a theory put forth by Frigyes Karinthy and made popular by a play written by John Guare, everyone is six or fewer steps away, by way of introduction, from any other person in the world. This is called **Six Degrees of Separation.** It literally means we can connect ourselves to anyone in six relationships or steps. (You know Joanne, who knows Marcy, who knows Gale, who knows Oprah, and on it goes.) Pretty cool, huh?

So if this is true, we are already connected to someone who can lead us to the people with whom we can share Community.

The concept of beginning a conversation with someone sounds simple, but sometimes it can actually feel difficult or overwhelming.

If you look at the funnel chart on page 129 and feel like you are hunting for a needle in a haystack, I'm here to remind you that <u>you are not</u>. Your job is just to begin talking about what you want and allow others to find you. The previous exercises in this Guidebook are key to that sharing.

Begin by telling your family, friends, co-workers and acquaintances that you are interested in forming and living in Community. (This step is surprisingly overlooked!) Never underestimate that someone you know right now may themselves be interested in Community or directly know someone who is. Make a list of the 10 to 30 people you talk to, see or correspond with every week. Then go back in a month or so and do it again. I promise your list will astound you.

Some examples to prime the pump:
- Your sister or brother
- The person who makes your coffee at the local coffee shop
- Your current neighbors
- You fitness instructor
- Your granddaughter's piano teacher
- People at your church, synagogue or mosque

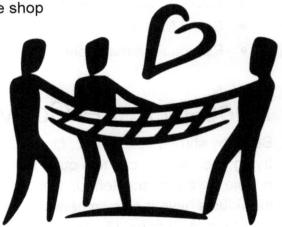

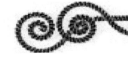 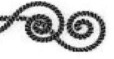

Exercise:

Now it's your turn. Write a list of the people in your life who you communicate with each week:

1.	9.
2.	10.
3.	11.
4.	12.
5.	13.
6.	14.
7.	15.
8.	16.

Now, take the next step and make sure these people learn about your Quest for Community. Don't let that Fire-Breathing Dragon of Distraction pull your attention somewhere else. Make a plan RIGHT NOW to send out an email, make a phone call or have a face-to-face with the people who you already know.

Social Media:

Today almost all of us are linked somehow to some form of social media. At the time of the writing of this Guidebook, Facebook®, Google+ ®, Twitter® and LinkedIn® are online Communities that almost everyone participates in somehow. Collecting "friends", and finding and cultivating Community is what social media was invented for. Inform your network about what's going on with you. You can make posts, give updates, engage in conversation and advertise meetings. Remember, because most social media is just a way to let people know your status, you can use it as a way of checking in and advertising for other like-minded Community seekers.

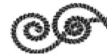
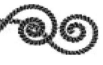

Here are a few sample posts that might stir some interest.

> *"I have decided I want to live in intentional community. This means I want to live with others to share expense, find security and cultivate relationships. I'm always open to talking to others who are interested in community."*

> *"I've just received my copy of "Your Quest for Home", a Guidebook to help me define how I want to live out my later years. I can't wait to dig in."*

> *"I've always loved the TV show "The Golden Girls". Are you or someone you know interested in living like those ladies?"*

> *"I am feeling so powerful because I am taking real action to determine how I want to live my later years. No Nursing Home for me!"*

Placing Ads:

Sometimes the best way to get the word out is the old fashioned way . . . placing an ad. You can put a short ad in a community newspaper or neighborhood circulars advertising meet and greet opportunities to talk about Community. Many papers (and their online versions) allow you to place these kinds of ads for free. You can also use social media as described previously as a means to get your advertising out there.

Don't forget to put up the tried and true flyer. People still look at community bulletin boards so create a flyer to place there. You can find these kinds of bulletin boards in local grocery stores, coffee shops, retail stores, libraries and community centers.

The Importance of Being Specific

Chances are, if you have worked through many of the exercises in this Guidebook, you have more clarity about what you are looking for. Use this information when you are throwing out your net and drumming up interest. It's critical to be as specific as possible.

If you state only that you want to live in Community, almost every person you talk to will visualize something different. So instead say things such as, "I'm looking to live with other single, retired women in a shared house." Or "I want to find a group of people who want to purchase homes near one another and form a supportive Community together as we get older." To do this, refer to some of the questions you have answered earlier in this Guidebook, especially your list of "Absolutely Must Haves".

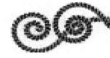 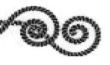

Travel Log

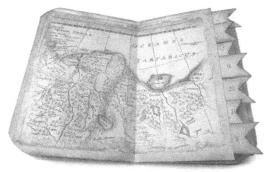

Use this space to organize information from the previous exercises, create to-do lists, and/or brainstorm the actions you want to take. Be sure to date your entries.

"If we go down into
ourselves we find that
we possess exactly
what we desire. "
                    Simone Weil

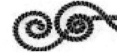
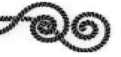

INVITE PEOPLE TO THE TABLE

Providing an Opportunity to Talk
About Community

Whether you are talking to people one-on-one or hosting gatherings of many people, the purpose of this next step is to begin conversations about your ideal Community and to find others who have a similar vision.

This will likely look different each time you do it. Most people you meet will not have given a lot of thought about living in Community. Then again others you meet may have been thinking and planning for years. You will have to deal with people all over the continuum.

Either way, the purpose of these interactions is to meet like-minded people no matter where they are in the process.

One-On-One Interactions:

One of the most common ways you will have these interactions will be one-on-one. You may go out for coffee or tea with someone you meet to share ideas and get to know one another. You may have conversations via email. Whatever the mechanism, the purpose quite simply is to begin getting to know one another and to determine if you want to continue the conversation.

141

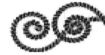
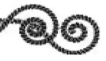

But what if you meet people you don't really connect with? That's okay. In fact, if you connected and actually wanted to live with everyone you met, that would be worrisome. This is a discernment process. Again, let's go back to the dating analogy. You can go out and have a great time with a lovely person but still not want to marry them, right? Same thing here.

What may happen is you begin connecting people to one another. As you begin to meet people who are also interested in Community, you will be able to connect them to others who want similar things, even if they don't want what you want. Connection at its best!

Community Potlucks/Gatherings:

One of the most effective (and frankly, the most fun and fruitful) means of throwing out the net is by hosting Community gatherings and potlucks. These can range in size and focus. You can have 3 or 4 people over for dinner at your house, or a gathering of up to 50 people at a community park.

The goal is to bring together people in person, who identify as being interested in Community. Setting the intention and the purpose of the gathering will help determine who will show up.

A couple of tips on bringing people together:

1. Choose a date that does not coincide with other major community events that might compete for people's attention.
2. Pick a time of day that would allow for the most people to attend. It has been my experience that late afternoon/early evening on a Saturday or Sunday works well for many people.
3. Give clear directions on how to get to the gathering. A map, directions and a phone number are essential.
4. Be very, VERY clear about the purpose of the meeting.
   a. "To meet other people who are considering living in a shared house."
   b. "To bring together people who want to start and build a neighborhood in the Chilhowee Neighborhood."
   c. "To bring together women in their 60's who want to talk about growing older and sharing housing."
5. Have a clear agenda with times that you, the host, follow and can share with the participants upon arrival.
6. Begin and end on time. If you want to extend the time you can, but make sure to have completed all the things on the agenda by the stated end time. This way people can leave and not feel like they are missing out on any content.

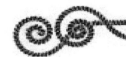
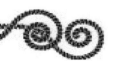

7. Gather contact information during the meeting.
8. GET PERMISSION FROM EVERYONE if you are going to share people's personal information or share pictures of the group.

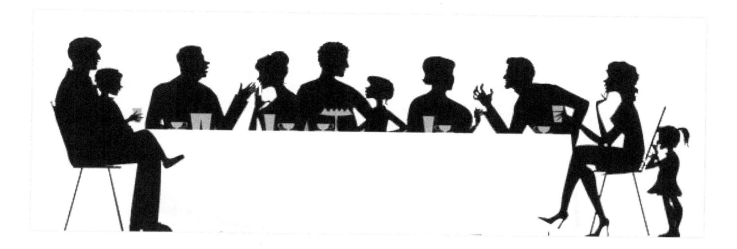

We've Gathered, Now What?

First, let's review why we have gathered people together in the first place . . . YOU WANT TO LIVE WITH AND AROUND OTHERS. Right? So to do this you have to meet and talk to a lot of people. You wouldn't settle down with the first woman or man you dated, would you?

There are many benefits of these interactive gatherings. First, we are all greater than the sum of our parts. Anytime people come together, new exciting ideas emerge. Secondly, everyone has unique gifts, ideas and networks, that when combined, can move a project along rather quickly. And lastly its fun (and it's Community!) One of the primary reasons a person wants to live in Community is to build relationships and feel supported. And that feeling can begin, right from the start.

In the next section there are tips about doing just that!

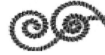
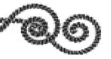

"Tell me, what is it you plan to do
with your one wild and precious life?"

Mary Oliver

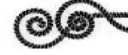
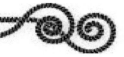

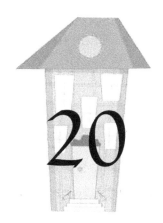

FIND COMMON GROUND

Gain a Deeper Understanding of One Another

Chances are you have met people who want to build Community with you.
Now what do you do?

Below are some ideas for activities and questionnaires that you can use to deepen your knowledge of one another and to determine if your goals are similar enough to proceed. *Note: I suggest everyone use this Guidebook. It will be a great way to get to know one another and stay focused.*

Building a Group

In the previous chapter there was a list of tips for gathering people together. Here is a list of ideas of things you can do as you get to know each other better.

Establish Shared Understanding

To really stretch and grow, one has to feel safe. This is especially true when we are asking ourselves and others to open our hearts. So that we can work smoothly with one another and create the safest space possible, we need to create a list of Shared Understandings.

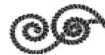
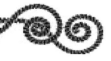

It is best to begin the discussion with a question such as "What rules or Shared Understandings do we want to follow during our meetings?" Then record the list on a shared space document or flipchart paper.

Examples:

> 1. Everyone speak for themselves using "I" statements.
>
> 2. No side conversations. It makes it difficult for everyone to hear.
>
> 3. Be respectful of and to one another.
>
> 4. Agree to disagree.
>
> 5. Honor the time.
>
> 6. Share the floor, and monitor how much you talk in comparison to others.
>
> 7. Honor confidentiality if someone shares something personal and private.

These are just suggestions. If you use these kinds of Shared Understandings from the beginning of your time together it will prevent many disagreements down the road.

Asking Questions

Asking and answering questions is one of the best ways to get to know others. The facilitator's job is to allow everyone to speak, share the space, keep the questions on topic and keep the event light and fun.

Start by picking fairly simple, non-threatening questions. I suggest you peruse this Guidebook and use some of the questions I have asked.

Here are a few basic questions to get things started:

1. Why do you want to live in Community?
2. What are three characteristics of your ideal living environment?
3. When you think about living with others, what excites you the most?
4. What are the gifts you can bring to a Community?

Group Activities

On the next few pages are some suggested exercises. You can duplicate and use them when you gather people together. Discussing individuals' answers can be a great jumping off point to facilitate rich discussions.

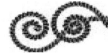
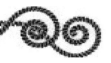

What Does Community Mean To Me?

Below is an activity you can use at a meeting. Read through it, use it as is or adapt it to meet your needs. Choose someone to facilitate this activity. It does not necessarily have to be you. Read aloud the following:

> "Sift back through your life, remembering times when you experienced Community in a powerful and profoundly meaningful way. Recall a time when you felt most alive in a Community; perhaps a time when you were most involved or most excited about your involvement. Choose one of these times to write about."

- What made this an exciting experience for you?

- Why is it you still remember this experience?

- Who else was with you? What were the qualities of those who made those relationships work?

- What were the VALUES that were shared or expressed in this experience?

- What did you take from this experience that applies to your current life?

- What was transformative about this experience?

147

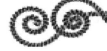
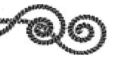

Group Activity

Who Am I?

Who Am I? is an activity that can be used to help individuals get to know themselves on a deeper level, and if the answers shared, get know others in the group.

You will need the following:

- A piece of paper for each person
- Index cards
- Name Tags
- Optional: an easel and flip chart

Follow steps 1 through 6 as they are written below. Be sure to allow discussion because this is often where the real learning happens.

Step 1: Make a short list of the names of individuals you admire. A person qualifies whether you know them personally or not, whether they are living or dead, or historical or fictional. Each must possess qualities you value or attributes you may wish for yourself.

Step 2: Next to each name, write down three of the qualities you admire in the person. These qualities can be one or two word phrases such as trustworthy, joy-filled, risk taker, etc. It might look like the example below.

NAME	QUALITIES/ATTRIBUTES		
Superman	Strength	Loyalty	Vision

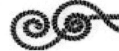
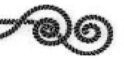

Step 3: Look at your list of Qualities/Attributes and see what, if any, themes emerge. Circle up to 5 themes that you might notice. Themes would be phrases that repeat on your list or are similar in meaning to you. For example: Being of service, great sense of humor, committed to learning, etc.

Step 4: Transfer your list of qualities/attributes onto an index card.

"This is who I have come here to be . . ."

Step 5: Ask each participant to choose the 3 most important qualities and legibly write them on their nametag.

Step 6: Circulate around the room and find others with similar qualities and attributes that match yours. Then talk about that !

Step 7: Discuss the following questions with the group.

- What did you learn about yourself when you chose the people you most admire?

- What themes emerged as you wrote down and studied the attributes of these people?

- What did you notice as you walked around and spoke with one another?

- Because you have identified these 3 attributes that are important to you, how might things change in your life?

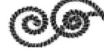
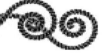

Group Activity

Reflections

Adapted from an exercise conducted at the Envisioning Home Conference 2013

1. Describe the physical place you <u>currently</u> refer to as "home." Is it an apartment, single family, shared housing?

2. What it is about this place that makes it "home" to you?

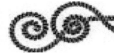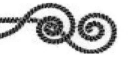

3. Imagine yourself having one of the life-changing events below.

    - rheumatoid or osteoarthritis
    - retirement or loss of a job
    - the loss of a spouse/partner (if you have one) through death, separation or divorce
    - moving from your home

    How would this event impact your current life and living situation?

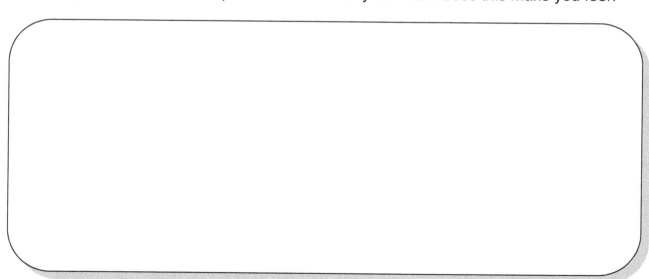

4. What do your answers to the questions above tell you? How does this make you feel?

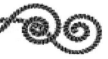

And a few more questions:

1. What are some of the reasons you want to live with or in proximity to others – women, men, families?

2. What stops you or might stop you from moving forward with this dream of living in Community?

3. What might help you to move forward? Is there something that you need to learn? What resources, skills or assistance might you need?

4. How can you prepare to move toward your dreams/vision/idea? What could be your next steps in moving forward?

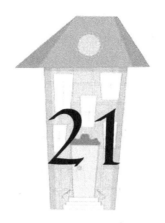

IDENTIFY MEMBERS OF YOUR COMMUNITY

Determine if Moving Forward is a Good Idea

How do you know if you want to move forward with a specific group of people?
The answer is **"When you know!"**

Let me ask you, how did you know which college you wanted to attend? Who you wanted to date, marry or start a business with? Which job offer to accept? Well, the process is the same. You use and TRUST your brain, your gut and your heart.

Using all three is your best bet for making choices that will serve your highest good. So if all three of these are in alignment, there is a pretty good chance you'll move forward. But in truth . . . this is hard to explain and sometimes even harder to do. Ultimately you will have to make your best guess and then diligently watch for clues and cues that you made the right choice.

Let's assume you have done many of the steps I have recommended so far. You have met one or more people who are possibilities for your Community and now you want to go deeper with this person. Remember, at the beginning, I told you that you would be asked to share your ideas for what you want with others? Now is the time.

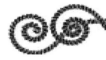
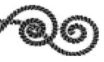

The challenge may be that many of the people you meet will not have given this journey as much thought as you have. This means you may find yourself walking them through many of the assessments you have already done. But have no fear . . . that's where this Guidebook comes in!

In addition to all the exercises you have already done, this chapter has a few more activities and worksheets to use when you are gathered with potential Community members.

The Importance of Good Communication

Clarity is the solution to almost any problem or challenges that will come up. Therefore being clear in all areas of your communication is a must. It is important to be very, VERY clear on your goals, your personal timeline, your finances, your "yes's" and "no's." It all begins with self-awareness and a willingness to say "yes" to what you want and "no" to what you don't want.

All of us can benefit and move forward when our written and verbal communication follows the Seven C's of Communication:

- Clear
- Concise
- Concrete
- Correct
- Coherent
- Complete
- Courteous

You DO NOT want to go further with someone who does not have clarity. Believe me!

Indications You Are Right for Each Other

- Your **values are in alignment**.
- Your desires are **compatible** or similar enough to move forward.
- You share a **similar timeline** for when you want to be in Community.
- You have or can **agree on a system for making decisions**.
- Once you live together, your **personal schedules will not conflict**.
- You **share the same level of passion** and intensity about this project and about life.
- You have **similar/compatible styles of communication**.
- You **agree on how often to communicate** with each other and the form it takes.
- You have **predetermined how you will settle a disagreement**.
- Your personal **habits do not overly annoy** one another.

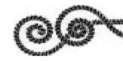
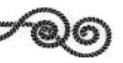

Do you have more considerations? If so, write them down below.

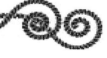

Group Activity

Community Readiness Questionnaire

Below are some questions to get you to begin thinking about living in Community. It is a comprehensive view that asks you to consider many different aspects of Community. Sit with the questions for a moment or two before writing your answers. After answering them ask yourself , "Am I ready?"

1.   What are some of the reasons you want to live with others?

2.   Describe how you might feel if you found and lived in the perfect Community?

3.   What might help you move forward?

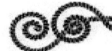
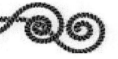

4. What might hold you back?

5. What resources, skills or assistance might you need?

6. Where would you like your Community to be?

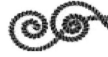
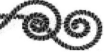

7. Who you would like to live with/near?

8. When or how soon are you ready to commit to moving?

9. Why do you want to do this?

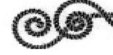
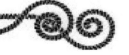

10. What could stop you from moving forward with this dream/vision?

11. Do you want to rent or buy? Why?

12. What type of Community model do you want to live in? Village, cohousing, shared housing or a combination. Or some other model?

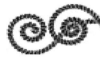
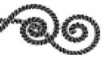

13. What is your financial situation? For example, are you pre-qualified for a home, do you have equity, are you retired with resources, etc.?

14. Which of the items below would you be willing to share? Not willing to share? Place a "Y" for Yes and an "N" for No.

_____ House	_____ Bathroom	_____ Housecleaning
_____ Car	_____ Computer	_____ Food
_____ Kitchen	_____ Yard tools	_____ Meals
_____ Books	_____ Yard work	_____ Other

15. How much space do you think you will need/want?

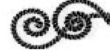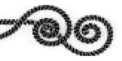

16. What is holding you back or what could hold you back from making a commitment?

_____ Money

_____ Time

_____ Fear of _____

_____ Getting rid of all my "stuff" such as _____

_____ Finding others to live in my Community _____

_____ The "right" place _____

_____ Taking too long _____

_____ Too many meetings to get there _____

_____ Am I really ready for this type of situation now _____

_____ My partner _____

_____ I had a bad experience with Community building and it is still with me

_____ Other: _____

If you are not ready yet, what actions do you need to take? For example, get your finances in order, call Marianne or read a book about Community.

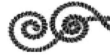
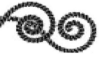

Personality Assessment & Group Building Tools

Understanding other humans has been a challenge since the beginning of time. Fortunately some easily accessible tools have been created to help us know ourselves and others better. Below I have highlighted just a few I have found helpful and which are fairly easy for groups to use. These modalities have undergone a lot of research and have stood the test of time as predictors of behavior and personality traits.

Here are just a few.

Myers Briggs™:

The Myers Briggs Type Indicator (MBTI) is a personality inventory that was developed by Isabel Briggs Myers, building on the work of C.G. Jung. His theory was that the personality traits that we have may seem random but in reality there is a real order to them. This is due to the different ways individuals use their perception and judgment.

The work puts forth four different aspects of one's life to examine:
- Do you prefer to focus on an inner world or an outer world? This is called Extraversion (E) or Introversion (I).
- Do you prefer to focus on basic information or to interpret information and add meaning to it? This is called Sensing (S) or Intuition (N).
- Do you make decisions from a place of logic or from a place of feeling? This is called Thinking (T) or Feeling (F).
- Do you like decisions to be clearly made or to remain open to new information coming in? This is called Judging (J) or Perceiving (P).

ISTJ	ISFJ	INFJ	INTJ
ISTP	ISFP	INFP	INTP
ESTP	ESFP	ENFP	ENTP
ESTJ	ESFJ	ENFJ	ENTJ

Each person has a preference in each of the above aspects. This means there are 16 different combinations. (For example: ISTJ or ENFP) Each of these personality types have a certain way they move through and perceive the world and all types are equal. Knowing how you perceive and judge the world can be incredibly helpful. It is very helpful if everyone in a group that plans to work together has this understanding as well.

For more information, begin at www.humanmetrics.com. There are lots of resources should this interest you.

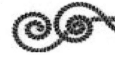
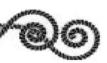

DISC™:

The DISC™ assessment is a behavior assessment based on the work of psychologist William Martst. His work centered around four different personality traits: Dominance, Inducement, Submission and Compliance. It was later developed into a personality assessment tool.

(Note: The words assigned to the letters "D" "I" "S" "C" have changed but the meaning still remain. It is thought that each of us have a preferred way of acting in the world.)

D: Dominance . . . this is an emphasis on overcoming opposition in your environment to get the results you want.

I: Influence . . . this is an emphasis on influencing or persuading others to shape your environment.

S: Steadiness . . . this is an emphasis on cooperating with others to get things done or accomplish a task.

C: Consciousness . . . this is an emphasis on working conscientiously within the specific circumstance to ensure quality and accuracy.

Like the Myers Briggs, there is a lot of information about this Personality Assessment Tool in books and on the Internet. You can begin your search to learn more at www.iscpersonalitytesting.com.

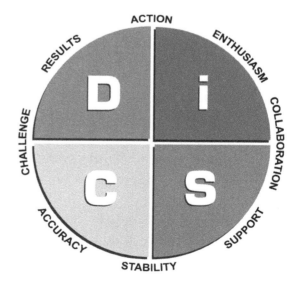

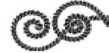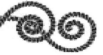

Enneagram:

The Enneagram is another personality typing system that consists of 9 different types. This system traces back to the Sufis and emerging information from modern day interests enhance its usefulness.

The nine types are identified by number and are placed around the Enneagram symbol. Each personality type has predictable behaviors, fears and ways to perceive the world that are unique to them. There are various others nuances to this modality. It is quite a detailed approach to personality typing and can be very profound and insightful.

Below are the nine types as described by Riso and Hudson. The names change a bit from writer to writer but the overall description of the various types remains consistent.

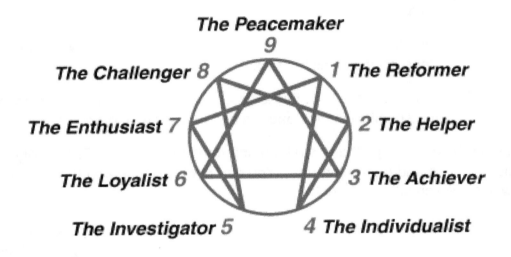

People of a particular type have several characteristics in common, but they can be quite different as well. There are a lot of different variables at play such as their level of mental health. Unhealthy people of a specific type can look very different from a healthy person with the same personality type. For this reason the Enneagram is not a parlor game but rather a serious study into how people think, feel and act.

This system is largely taught through self-disclosure. If you ever get a chance to attend a workshop, it could be helpful to your journey.

Begin your search here at www.enneagraminstitute.com where there is more information available.

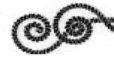
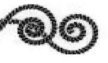

Astrology:

Whether you believe in astrology or not, it is a timeless way of looking at yourself and your personality and proclivity.

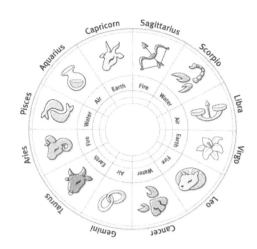

It is a system based on a relationship between the alignment of the planets at the time of your birth. The most common way people use astrology is through horoscopes but there is much more to this modality. Many cultures use astrology in some form. The Indians, the Chinese and the Mayans have developed elaborate systems to study and use the planets as predictors and guides. There are many sites online to give you information about your sign.

It takes all types. These and other personality typing methods allow you to give and get information quickly about others in your group as it is forming. Using one of these methods is a suggested way to assist in the "culling" process of finding our Community members.

As you learn about yourself, you can have in-depth conversations and provide some insights into who you are according to these typing methods.

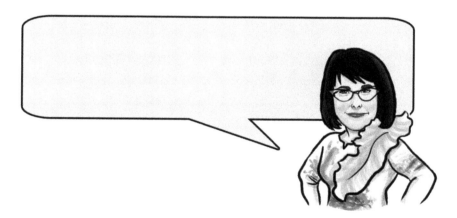

For example: You could be an ENFJ in the Myers Briggs (which is extrovert, intuitive, feeling oriented and organized person who is also a Scorpio and has the coping strategy of the 4 on the Enneagram and is a "D" on the Disc. What would this tell someone about you?

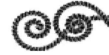
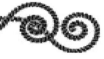

"Community
means that we
have a place
where we belong
no matter who
we are."
Hilary Clinton

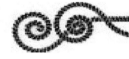
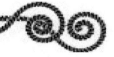

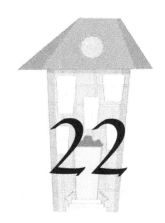

TAKE ACTION WITH YOUR COMMUNITY

Deciding How to Move Forward To Form "Your" Community

This Guidebook is about your Quest. More resources are becoming available for you all the time. Here are theories from experts about how we work together as a group of humans coming together. Being aware of them may allow you to relax and know that the stages are part of the process and to be expected when they show up. This is a small taste of the information about group formation.

Forming, Storming, Norming

There is a plethora of information out there about how groups come together and form into a lasting, vibrant, healthy union . . . or ultimately blow up. Depending on what you read, you will find variations on the number of stages a group goes through. But many of these researchers say the same thing. Groups go through particular stages and often have particular behavior as they mature.

The Forming, Storming, Norming and Performing model of group development was developed by Bruce Tuckerman in 1965. He stated that these stages were NECESSARY and inevitable for a team (and that would mean Community too) to grow and effectively face challenges. Many people have built on this work and added more stages, but let's use Tuckerman's work to get started.

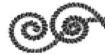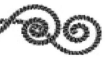

Forming:

This stage is where all groups begin. People in the group are typically unclear about their roles and responsibilities. The group is just beginning to define its purpose and what it hopes to accomplish. In this stage the members rely heavily on the guidance of the leader. (A real challenge if there isn't one!)

Storming:

Every group goes through the storming phase because this is when various ideas compete for consideration. This is also when problems make themselves known and people within the group have different ideas of how to approach these problems. This is a necessary stage of development because a lot of things float to the surface and many strategies and decisions are made for how to deal with problems in the future. Not all team members "survive" this stage. In others words, some folks may decide to pull out. But that's okay. Those who remain have a deeper understanding of one another and the purpose of the group.

Norming:

It's at this point that the group has agreed upon a goal and a plan for making that goal a reality. Some people of the group may have had to give up their personal preference so the group can function. But all of the team members take responsibility and have a vision of success. Groups have to be careful in this stage because people within the group may stop sharing their different viewpoints for fear of rocking the boat.

Performing:

Some very hardworking and lucky groups reach the performing state. These groups can function as one to get things done smoothly and effectively without conflict (or much anyway). Everyone knows what their responsibilities are and takes care of them. The group members are autonomous and can make decisions on their own that serve the whole. Disagreements are allowed as long as they are resolved through the process which the group has set up.

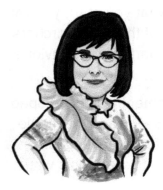

Note: Movement through these stages is not a linear or sequential process. Groups can go forward, skip steps entirely or even go backwards. It's okay and a part of this natural process.

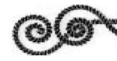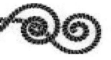

TRUTH IN PARTNERING, FULL DISCLOSURE
A Basis for Conscious Community building

The following is an in-depth questionnaire to be used to summarize previous exercises in this Guidebook or used as a intense stand-alone exercise. This tool is offered to us by a friend and fellow communitarian, Carol Pimenthal.

<u>You and You</u>

1. What individual visions, dreams and goals do you have for your life? When you come to the end of your life and look back, what will make you feel that you made the most of your time on earth?
   - Purpose, mission, context for your life, if you are aware of one
   - Important values & qualities you want to embody and live from
   - Experiences you want to have, contributions you want to make
   - Where and how you want to live
   - Describe the factors of a rich, vibrant life with you thriving. What lights you up?

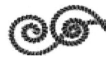

2. What are you up to now, with timetables if any, and what is the bigger picture for this activity? (e.g. I'm focused on school now, which will take me 5 years, with the intention of becoming able to support my family by doing what I love, and make a valuable contribution to society.)

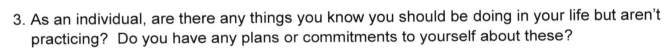

3. As an individual, are there any things you know you should be doing in your life but aren't practicing? Do you have any plans or commitments to yourself about these?

You and Community

4. What do you see as the gains and the losses for you as you get involved in long-term Community building and Community membership?

5. In a Community relationship:
- What purpose does/will Community serve in your life?
- What are you in it for; what do you expect/hope to get; what will you ask of others?
- What do you have to offer; what do you expect to give or provide to the group?
- What do you perceive to be your own liabilities, vulnerabilities or weaknesses as a Community member?
- Do you have any commitments or plans to change or grow in these areas?
- What "baggage" do you bring from your past that might cause some problems?

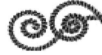
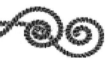

6. Your Community vision:
   a. In a series of short sentences, describe all the important elements of fulfilling, inspiring Community living *for you.* These are your deepest wishes and dreams for fulfillment in Community living.

   b. What purpose would the Community have, if any, beyond mutual enjoyment? How do you envision the group serving or participating in the larger Community?

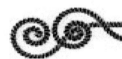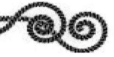

c. What key values would be shared by your Community? How would these show up in daily living?

d. What physical elements are important to you in a Community: location, geography, climate, building style, aesthetics, energy efficiency? What bottom line elements could you not compromise on?

e. What facilities and decisions would be shared, and what would be private?

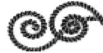

"If what's in your dreams wasn't already real inside you, you couldn't even dream it."

Gloria Steinem

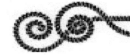
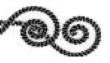

23

Resources

Organizations/Networks

Beacon Hill Village – a neighborhood-created-without-walls retirement community in central Boston that partners with service providers to offer its paying members access to social and cultural activities, exercise opportunities, household and home maintenance services. www.beaconhillvillage.org

Center for Collaborative Awareness offers tools for creating healthier, more adaptable collaborations at work and at home. www.blueprintofwe.com

Center for Non Violent Communication is a global organization that helps people peacefully and effectively resolve conflicts in personal, organizational, and political settings. www.cnvc.org

Communities Magazine – The primary resource for information, issues, stories and ideas about intentional communities in North America—from urban co-ops to cohousing groups to ecovillages and rural communes. www.communities.ic.org

ElderSpirit Community – Located in Abingdon, VA, is a unique intentional community that has combined many components in such a way that a lifestyle for pro-active elders has purpose and meaning. www.elderspirit.org

Golden Girls Network – A supportive and nurturing network which improves the quality of life and enhances self-reliance for single mature women and men by connecting them through shared living and social networking. www.goldengirlsnetwork.org

Governance Alive – Dynamic Governance is a decision-making and governance model that rewires the decision-making process. www.governancealive.com/dynamic-governance

Fellowship of Intentional Communities (FIC) – The Fellowship for Intentional Community nurtures connections and cooperation among communitarians and their friends. www.fic.ic.org

Let's Share Housing – Primarily based in Portland, Oregon, serving the Metro Portland area, the site helps members nationwide find one another by providing resources and links to other home sharing services. www.letssharehousing.com

National Shared Housing Resource Center – A clearinghouse of information for people looking to find a shared housing organization in their community or to help get a program started. www.nationalsharedhousing.org

NCB Capital Impact – THE GREEN HOUSE® Project provides technical assistance and partners with the lending team of Capital Impact to explore financing vehicles to organizations that want to establish THE GREEN HOUSE® homes. www.ncbcapitalimpact.org/home/expert-technical-assistance/green-house/

Rasur Foundation International – Teaches BePeace, a synergistic skill set for building social and emotional intelligence. www.rasurinternational.org

Second Journey – Mindfulness, Service and Community in the Second Half of Life. www.secondjourney.org

The Cohousing Association – Cohousing is a type of collaborative housing in which residents actively participate in the design and operation of their own neighborhoods. Cohousing residents are consciously committed to living as a community. http://www.cohousing.org

The Elder Cohousing Network – The Elder Cohousing Network provides helpful resources to support pro-active adults in creating their own intentional elder neighborhood. www.abrahampaiss.com/ElderCohousing

The Sage-ing Guild – The Sage-ing Guild is an association of individuals who share a passion for helping themselves and others age consciously. www.sage-ingguild.org.

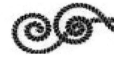
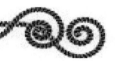

The Transition Network – An inclusive community of professional women, 50 and forward, whose changing life situations lead them to seek new connections, resources, and opportunities. www.TheTransitionNetwork.org

Village to Village Network – VtV helps communities establish and manage their own Villages. www.vtvnetwork.org

Women for Living in Community – Advocating for alternative housing choices as we age to share information, form connections and take action. Founder Marianne Kilkenny offers coaching, speaking, workshops, and resources. www.womenforlivingincommunity.com

Books

Blanchard, Janice. *Aging in Community Revised Edition.* Chapel Hill: Second Journey Press, 2013.

Block, Peter. *Community: The Structure of Belonging.* San Francisco: Berrett-Koehler, 2008.

Bolen, Jean Shinoda. *Crones Don't Whine.* Boston: Conari Press, 2003.

Buck, John and Sharon Villines. *We the People, A Guide to Sociocratic Principles and Method.* Washington D.C.: Sociocracy info Press, 2007.

Bush, Karen, Louise Machinist and Jean McQuillin. *My House Our House: Living Far Better for Far Less in a Cooperative Household.* Pittsburgh: St. Lynn's Press, 2013.

Carnes, Robin Deen and Sally Craig. *Sacred Circles, A Guide to Creating Your Own Women's Spirituality Group.* New York: Harper SanFrancisco, 1998.

Chiras, Dan and Dave Wann. *Superbia! 31 Ways to Create Sustainable Neighborhoods.* Gabriola Island, BC: New Society Publishers, 2003.

Christian, Diana Leafe. *Creating a Life Together: Practical Tools to Grow Ecovillages and Intentional Communities.* Gabriola Island, BC: New Society Publishers, 2003.

Christian, Diana Leafe. *Finding Community: How to Join an Ecovillage or Intentional Community.* Gabriola Island, BC: New Society Publishers, 2007.

Cohen, Gene, MD, PhD. *The Creative Age: Awakening Human Potential in the Second Half of Life.* New York: Avon Books, 2000.

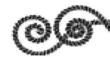
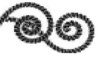

Dass, Ram. *Still Here: Embracing Aging, Changing and Dying*. New York: Penguin Books, 2000.

Durrett, Charles. *The Senior Cohousing Handbook: A Community Approach to Independent Living. 2nd edition.* Gabriola Island, BC: New Society Publishers, 2009.

Durrett, Charles. *Cohousing: A Contemporary Approach to Housing Ourselves*. Berkeley: Ten Speed Press, 1988.

Eiland, Natasha and Emmett Eiland. *The Last Resort.* Berkeley: Berkeley Hills Books, 2005.

Lawrence-Lightfoot, Sara. *The Third Chapter: Passion, Risk & Adventure in the 25 Years After 50*. New York: Sarah Crichton Books, 2009.

Leider, Richard, and David Shapiro. *Claiming Your Place at the Fire: Living the Second Half of Your Life on Purpose*. San Francisco: Berrett-Koehler Publishers, Inc., 2004.

Levine, Suzanne Braun. *Inventing the Rest of Our Lives*. New York: Penguin Books, 2006.

Luke, Helen. *Old Age: Journey into Simplicity*. Gt. Barrington MA: Lindisfarne Books, 2010.

Marohnm, Stephanie. *Audacious Aging.* Santa Rosa CA: Elite Books, 2009.

Mazer, Gwen with portraits by Christine Alicino. *Wise Talk, Wild Women*. San Francisco: Council Oak Books, 2007.

Medlicott, Joan. *The Ladies of Covington Series.* New York: Pocket Books.

Morgaine, Morgana. *Borderless Broads. New Adventures for the Midlife Woman*. DoneForYouPublishing.com, 2011.

Orsi, Janelle and Emily Drucker. *The Sharing Solution: How to Save Money, Simplify Your Life and Build Community*. Berkeley: Nolo Press, 2009.

Pipher, Mary PhD. *Another Country: Navigating the Emotional Terrain of Our Elders*. New York: Riverhead Books, 1999.

Pluhar, Annamarie. *Sharing Housing: A Guidebook for Finding and Keeping Good Housemates*. Peterborough NH: Bauhan Publishing, 2011.

Ruiz, Don Miguel. *The Four Agreements*. San Rafael CA: Amber-Allen Publishing, Inc., 1997 and 2012.

Sadler, William, PhD, and James Krefft, PhD. *Changing Course...Navigating Life After 50*. The

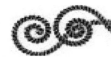
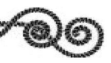

Center for Third Age Leadership Press, 2007.

Schachter-Shalomi, Zalman and Ronald Miller. *From Age-ing to Sage-ing: A New Vision of Growing Older.* New York: Warner Books, 1995.

Shaffer, Carolyn and Kristin Anundsen. *Creating Community Anywhere, Finding Support and Connection in a Fragmented World.* New York: Tarcher/Putnam, 1994.

Shapiro, Patricia Gottlieb. *Heart to Heart: Deepening Women's Friendships at Midlife.* Berkeley: Berkeley Books, 2001.

Thomas, William MD. *What are Old People For? How Elders Will Save the World.* Acton MA: VanderWyk and Burnham, 2004.

Wann, David. *Reinventing Community: Stories from the Walkways of Cohousing.* Golden, CO: Fulcrum Press, 2005.

Wheatley, Margaret. *Turning to One Another: Simple Conversations to Restore Hope to the Future.* San Francisco, Berrett-Koehler Publishers, Inc., 2009.

Online

Abrahms, Sally. "Elder Cohousing: A new option for retirement – or sooner!" *AARP Bulletin,* January 31, 2011. http://www.aarp.org/home-garden/housing/info-01-2011/elder_cohousing.1.html

Bennett, Ronni. Blog: *Time Goes By: What It's Really Like to Get Older.* http://www.timegoesby.net/

Bolstler, Heather. Blog: *Shedders.* http://shedders.wordpress.com/

Cicero, Dr. Caroline. "It Takes a Village." *Huff Post Post 50,* August 18, 2012. http://www.huffingtonpost.com/dr-caroline-cicero/village-movement_b_1794479.html

Colin, Chris. "To Your Left, A Better Way of Life?" *New York Times,* June 10, 2009. http://www.nytimes.com/2009/06/11/garden/11cohousing.html

Hindman, Susan. "Green Houses Offer Community to Elders." *Silver Planet,* Sept. 10, 2009. http://www.silverplanet.com/silver-planet-aging/green-houses-offer-Community-elders/55516

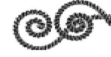
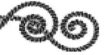

Hindman, Susan. "Housing Options: A Glossary – A Framework for Understanding Your Choices." *Silver Planet*, July 13, 2010. http://www.silverplanet.com/housing/housing-options-glossary/55728#.UkmmYq3D-po

Mahoney, Sarah. "The New Housemates." *AARP The Magazine*, July 2007. http://www.aarp.org/home-garden/housing/info-2007/the_new_housemates.html

Mandhana, Niharika. "Shared Meals, and Lives." *New York Times*, Sept 28, 2013. http://newoldage.blogs.nytimes.com/2011/08/22/shared-meals-and-lives/?_r=2#more-9999

Mawhinney, Alex. "Intentional Elder Neighborhoods." *Second Journey*. http://www.secondjourney.org/itin/2010Spr/Mawhinney_2010Spr.htm

Ruiz, Don Miguel. The Four Agreements. Online at: http://www.toltecspirit.com/

Thomas, William MD. Blog: ChangingAging: a multi-blog platform challenging conventional views on aging. www.changingaging.com

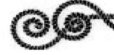
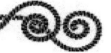

May the Road Rise Up to Meet You

Thanks for going on this Quest with me.

Your Quest has just begun . . .

There are many of us on this Quest, and some who don't know it yet . . . you are ahead of them . . . lead on . . . find others and we can change the face of aging as we move into our Second or Third part of life.

My hope is you are now equipped with ideas, insights, and illumination to light the path. Be fearless, don't give up—it's worth taking the next steps.

Marianne

Marianne Kilkenny

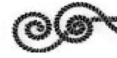
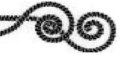

ACKNOWLEDGMENTS

To my collaborator in all things creative—the sassy coach and mentor Cheri Britton who always makes me look good.

To my housemates through the years who put up with me as I asked them to allow folks, including the national press, to wander through our house, asking questions about shared housing — and they just smiled. To the media for attention to Community and its importance in the lives of the Boomer Generation as a housing/living alternative that we are welcoming back again.

To "The Golden Girls" television show with those iconic ladies who showed us how to zestfully laugh, love and thrive in our later years.

To the wonderful Joan Medlicott and her Ladies of Covington series that attracted me to the mountains of North Carolina to live. She gave me permission to realize that her dream could be more than fiction.

To all of you who have attended my workshops, conferences, Meet Ups, talks, and seminars, or have talked to me on the phone, or allowed me to speak with passion about the concept of Aging in Community.

To that man who sat next to me many years ago at a National Speakers Association luncheon and said with a horrified look that no one would ever want to listen to a speaker talk about aging!

To my amazing clients who realized working together would be more fun and faster.

To the Women for Living in Community Meet Up in Asheville which has allowed me to flesh out my material with them, listen with attention and give feedback to the process.

To my loving sister, Madeline Lott for her gift with words as she helped me craft my message clearly. To Tena Frank, Vicky Goodridge and Susan Schankle for their attention to detail and kind manner in editing.

To those of you who called and said, "I don't want to live alone! What can I do?" and those of you who said, "Thanks for what you are doing, we need it." Your comments and encouragements have kept me charged up and inspired to do this important work.

To my colleagues who are adding to the work I started, adding resources, databases and more books and workshops to come.

Special thanks to Linda Williams, my Sarasota sister, who not only has helped me grow personally and professionally but has also encouraged and challenged me to pursue my dreams.

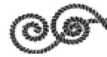
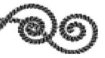

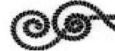
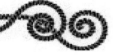

ABOUT THE AUTHOR

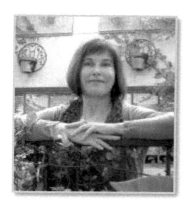

Marianne Kilkenny is the Trailblazer and the Grand Nudge behind the Women for Living in Community Network. She is a speaker and coach who works with individuals and groups to develop innovative models for living and aging in Community. She is a nationally recognized expert in shared homes and other forms of Community building and currently lives in a collaborative house in Asheville, North Carolina.

Her story has appeared in various media sources including NBC Nightly News, Good Morning America, More Magazine, WNC Woman, Smart Money, NPR, Reuters, and the AARP Bulletin. She has conducted numerous interviews for radio, print publications and blogs.

Marianne founded the Women for Living in Community Network in 2007 to work with individuals interested in changing the paradigm of aging. She encourages women to take the helm on projects to create Community living situations for themselves and others.

Marianne is a popular and engaging speaker and provides workshops throughout the US on topics such as *Aging in Community*, *Creating Community for the Second Half of Life*, and *A Solution to Bag Lady Fear Syndrome*.

The Grand Nudge, Marianne's alter ego, is the more direct side of her personality. The Grand Nudge's mission is to get you out of your seat so you can make Community happen NOW because no one is going to do it for you.

Prior to launching Women for Living in Community, Marianne worked for 25 years as a Human Resources Director in Silicon Valley. She earned her bachelor's degree in Management from California State University at Chico.

Marianne pulls from many resources, including her own life experience, when speaking and teaching about Community living. She is a Certified Senior Cohousing Facilitator and Trainer and also completed training in the Cohousing Development Process from the Elder Cohousing Network in Boulder, Colorado. While the most common form of Community living for women can be seen in the "Golden Girls" model, Marianne understands the wide varieties of options and can help individuals and groups explore the right ones for their own needs.

Marianne is actively enjoying a Community lifestyle and likes to share her story with anyone interested in pursuing the same for themselves. She has a zest for life and brings her sense of humor with her wherever she goes.

Learn more about Marianne's coaching, speaking and trailblazing
www.womenforlivingincommunity.com

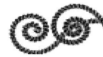
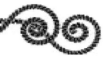

Marianne Kilkenny

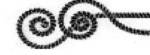
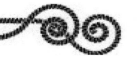

ABOUT THE EDITOR/DESIGNER

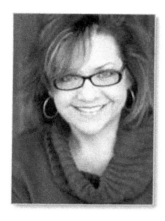

Cheri Britton is a Dynamite Motivational Speaker, Corporate Trainer and Effectiveness Coach. So why is she doing editing and designing this Guidebook? Because she can!

In addition to being a extraordinary speaker and coach she also loves to help others bring their ideas to fruition. In this case, she not only loves and respects Marianne and her mission but she believes the time has come for her important work to be put out into the world through this Guidebook.

She speaks nationally about getting unstuck—what she calls BOOM Thinking™ because she knows being stagnant leads to a lack-luster life. Her belief is that breaking free of our old worn-out beliefs facilitates us all to step into new actions. It is the combining of these new beliefs with solid, concrete actions that make us to happy, motivated and fired up. And let's be honest, who doesn't want that?!

She has written two books of her own, *"BOOM Thinking: The Gutsy Guide to Breaking Out of Old Mindsets"* and *"Work Your 'But' Off: A 30 Day Programs to Help You Eliminate Excuses and Get your Buts Off the Couch!"* Both can be found through her website or on Amazon.com.

Find out more about Cheri, her speaking topics, her products, or read her blog at **www.cheribritton.com.**

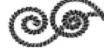

CPSIA information can be obtained
at www.ICGtesting.com
Printed in the USA
LVHW061615180319
610886LV00009B/7/P